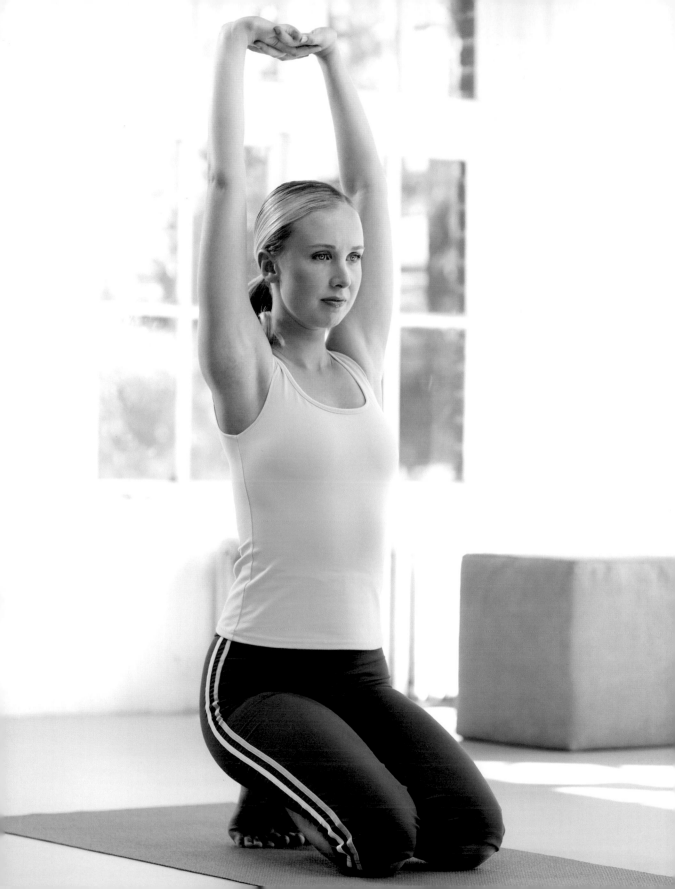

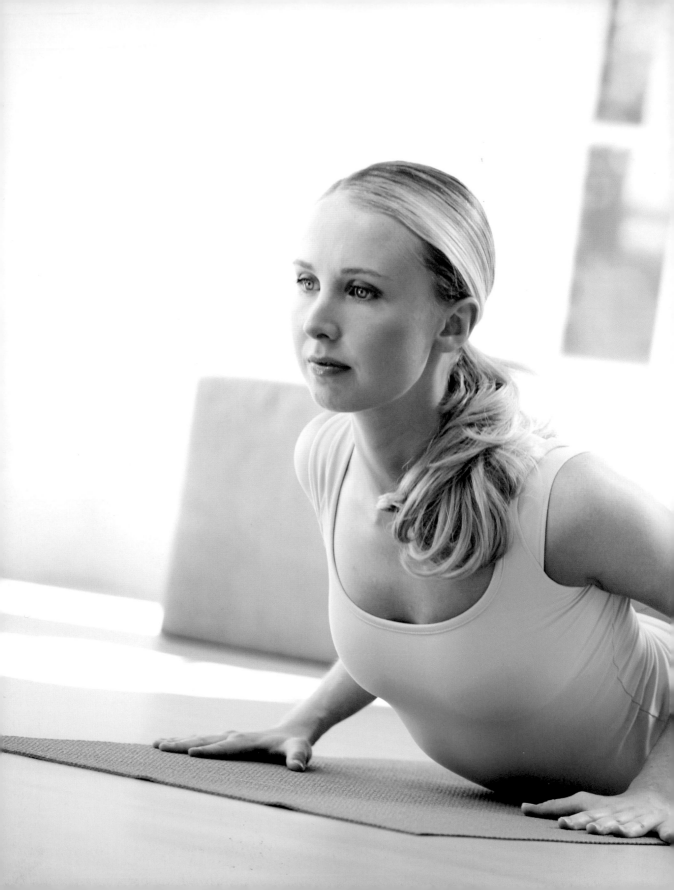

>> **15** minute gentle yoga

Louise Grime

London, New York, Melbourne, Munich, Delhi

Project Editor Helen Murray
Project Art Editor Anne Fisher
Senior Art Editor Peggy Sadler
Managing Editor Penny Warren
Managing Art Editor Marianne Markham
Art Director Peter Luff
Publishing Director Mary-Clare Jerram
Stills Photography Ruth Jenkinson
DTP Designer Sonia Charbonnier
Production Controller Rebecca Short
Production Editor Luca Frassinetti
Jacket Designer Neal Cobourne

DVD produced for Dorling Kindersley by
Chrome Productions www.chromeproductions.com

Director Sami Abusamra
DOP Marcus Domleo, Matthew Cooke
Camera Marcus Domleo, Jonathan Iles
Production Manager Hannah Chandler
Production Assistant Krisztina Fenyvesi, Tom Robinson
Grip Pete Nash
Gaffer Paul Wilcox, Johann Cruickshank
Music Chad Hobson
Hair and Makeup Roisin Donaghy, Victoria Barnes
Voice-over Suzanne Pirret
Voice-over Recording Ben Jones

First American Edition, 2008

Published in the United States by
DK Publishing
375 Hudson Street
New York, New York 10014

08 09 10 9 8 7 6 5 4 3

HD130-Jan 08

Copyright © 2008 Dorling Kindersley Limited
Text copyright © 2008 Louise Grime

Published in Great Britain by Dorling Kindersley Limited.

A catalog record for this book is available from the Library of Congress

ISBN 978-0-7566-2926-7

DK books are available at special discounts when purchased in bulk for sales promotions, premiums, fund-raising, or educational use. For details, contact: DK Publishing Special Markets, 375 Hudson Street, New York, New York 10014 or SpecialSales@dk.com.

Printed and bound by Sheck Wah Tong, China

Discover more at
www.dk.com

contents

Health warning
Always consult your doctor before starting a fitness program if you have any health concerns, and especially if you are pregnant, have given birth in the last six weeks, or have a medical condition such as high blood pressure, arthritis, or asthma. This book is not intended for people suffering from back problems; it provides programs to strengthen the back and prevent back problems from occurring. If you have any pain while exercising, stop immediately.

Every effort has been made to ensure that the information contained in this book is complete and accurate. However, neither the publisher nor the author is engaged in rendering professional advice or services to the individual reader. The ideas, information, and suggestions contained in this book are not intended as a substitute for consulting with your physician. All matters regarding your health require medical supervision. Neither the author nor the publisher shall be liable or responsible for any loss or damage allegedly rising from any information or suggestion in this book.

author foreword

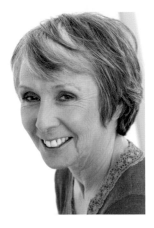

Yoga is truly amazing. It can wake you up to your true self, help you to let go of your preconditioned armor and to find inner joy. What more could you want?

When I was 27 years old, managing restaurants, I was lacking energy and I had no real passion in my life. I was just drifting along, smoking and drinking a little too much, and often at the doctor's office with niggling coughs. Then a friend sent me to a local yoga class and that was it. I knew from that very first class that I had fallen in love—fallen in love with the yogic journey of finding myself—and I want to share a little of that with you. The smoking and drinking just dropped away; I changed careers, becoming a stage manager in the theater, which then led to working in television production. I worked freelance and this enabled me to take several months off in between jobs. I went to the Sivananda Ashram (a country yoga center) in southern India to take a teachers' training course, not thinking I really wanted to teach, but for my own personal growth. I returned the following year, this time as a member of staff at the Ashram, immersing myself in all branches of yogic life from morning until night. I soon started teaching, and immediately loved it and converted the apartment above my home into a little yoga school. In the early 90's, I qualified as an Iyengar Yoga Teacher and this method has had the most influence on my practice and teaching. At that time I met the teacher who inspired me the most, Shandor Remete (Natanaga Zhander), who has now created Shadow Yoga. The Life Centre opened, and shortly afterward triyoga, the centers in London, where I teach. Slowly, I taught more and worked in television less. I have now taught for 19 years, and full-time for seven. I still love to learn from other teachers and go on yoga retreats and vacations, where you meet like-minded people from different walks of life.

***Gentle Yoga* contains four simple hatha yoga sequences**. You are asked to practice for just 15 minutes each day, but of course you can do more than that if you like. This book is designed to give you a taste of yoga and hopefully, like me, it will leave you wanting to learn more.

"Practice, and all is coming" K. Pattabhi Jois

Louise

>> **how to use** this book

Each sequence is designed to give you more energy, improve flexibility and posture, and to help ease the tension in your lives. Take time to study the poses in detail and familiarize yourself with what you will need to do. Use the gatefold summary as a quick reminder.

The accompanying DVD is designed to be used with the book to reinforce the exercises shown there. As you watch the DVD, page references to the book flash up on screen. Refer to these for more detailed instruction. In the book, the large photographs show the main pose. There are also inset photographs that are used in a number of ways: to show a starting position, a transitional pose, the next stage of the pose, or the pose from another angle. This is to make it clearer for you to follow and to ensure the sequence flows from one pose to another. Some poses are more difficult than others. The pink inset photographs indicate an easier option, where the pose is modified or props are added to make the pose more comfortable or simpler for beginners. The introductory pages, the FAQs (Frequently Asked Questions) at the end of each sequence, and the All About Yoga section provide further tips and information to enhance your practice.

The first poses in each sequence are warm-up and breathing exercises. The next are the main poses of the sequence, working the entire body. Finally, each sequence ends on a softer note, with the Final Relaxation.

The four sequences are intended for different parts of the day, but they work just as well at any time. Find a time that suits you best. They take 15 minutes each, but if you are a beginner, take as long as you need to learn the poses. For a longer practice, combine the sequences, omitting the final relaxation from each sequence until the very end.

The gatefold

The gatefold summaries at the end of each sequence help you to see each sequence in full view. Once you've watched the DVD and examined each pose, use the handy gatefolds as a quick reference to trim your practice down to a succinct 15 minutes.

energizer at a glance

1 ▲ Chin Mudra, page 70
2 ▲ Alternate Nostril Breathing, page 70
3 ▲ Kneeling Pose, Cow Face, page 71
4 ▲ Kneeling Pose, interlacing, page

13 ▲ Rest, page 76
14 ▲ Locust, page 76
15 ▲ Locust/Rest, page 77
16 ▲ Quadriceps Stretch, page 77

The gatefold gives you a comprehensive demonstration of the entire sequence—an easy reference to make your practice quick and simple.

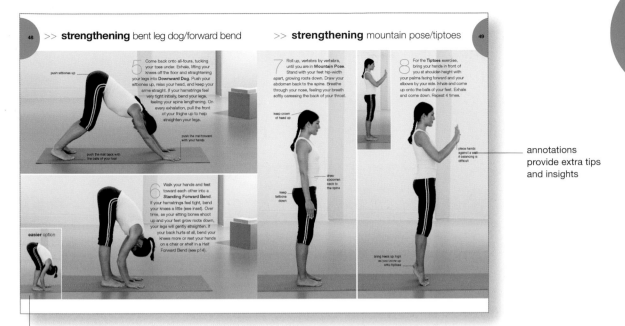

5 Come back onto all-fours, tucking your toes under. Exhale, lifting your knees off the floor and straightening your legs into **Downward Dog**. Push your sitbones up, relax your head, and keep your arms straight. If your hamstrings feel very tight initially, bend your legs, feeling your spine lengthening. On every exhalation, pull the front of your thigh up to help straighten your legs.

push sitbones up

push the mat forward with your hands

push the mat back with the balls of your feet

6 Walk your hands and feet toward each other into a **Standing Forward Bend**. If your hamstrings feel tight, bend your knees a little (see inset). Over time, as your sitting bones shoot up and your feet grow roots down, your legs will gently straighten. If your back hurts at all, bend your knees more or rest your hands on a chair or shelf in a Half Forward Bend (see p14).

easier option

7 Roll up, vertebra by vertebra, until you are in **Mountain Pose**. Stand with your feet hip-width apart, growing roots down. Draw your abdomen back to the spine. Breathe through your nose, feeling your breath softly caressing the back of your throat.

keep crown of head up

draw abdomen back to the spine

keep tailbone down

8 For the **Tiptoes** exercise, bring your hands in front of you at shoulder-height with your palms facing forward and your elbows by your side. Inhale and come up onto the balls of your feet. Exhale and come down. Repeat 4 times.

place hands against a wall if balancing is difficult

bring heels up high as you come up onto tiptoes

annotations provide extra tips and insights

pink inset photographs show the easier options, where the pose is modified or a prop is used

Step-by-step pages The large photographs show the main pose. The inset photographs indicate a starting position, a transitional movement, the next stage of the pose, or show the pose from another angle.

the gatefold shows all the main steps of the sequence

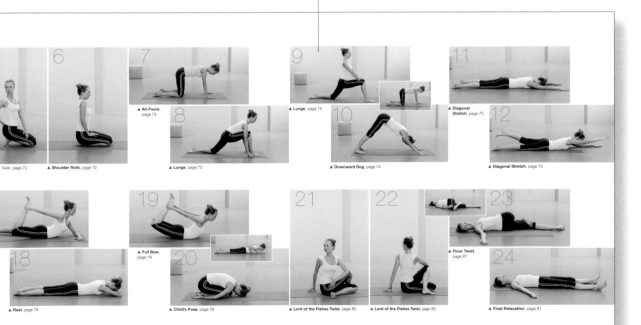

6

7

▲ All-Fours, page 73

8

9

▲ Lunge, page 74

10

11

▲ Diagonal Stretch, page 75

12

...ose, Twist, page 72   ▲ Shoulder Rolls, page 72

▲ Lunge, page 73

▲ Downward Dog, page 74

▲ Diagonal Stretch, page 75

18

19

▲ Full Bow, page 79

20

21

22

23

▲ Floor Twist, page 81

24

▲ Rest, page 78

▲ Child's Pose, page 79

▲ Lord of the Fishes Twist, page 80

▲ Lord of the Fishes Twist, page 80

▲ Final Relaxation, page 81

>> **introduction**

Welcome to yoga, whether you are trying it out to feel more fit and more flexible, or to de-stress and energize your mind and body. As you practice, you may find that yoga becomes a way of life and you start to approach every aspect of your day with an inquiring, balanced yoga mind-set.

When you embrace yoga, it becomes much more than what you do on the mat—it begins to filter into your way of thinking and interacting with others. As the postures and breathing practices make you feel bright and alive, so your self-confidence and energy levels soar; as you begin to notice where in the body you hold tension, and free it up by stretching and breathing more effectively, so you begin to become less stressed in your mind, too, and more able to appreciate life from different perspectives—just as yoga postures ask you to see the world upside down, backward, or sideways. As your physical balance improves, so does your ability to adopt a more measured approach to decision making and problem solving, enhancing every aspect of life, from your relationships at home and work to the way in which you do business. Above all, yoking together your body and mind with the single focus of a yoga posture makes every part of you feel more harmonious.

What is hatha yoga?

In the West, we tend to think of yoga as a system of physical exercises (known as *asanas*) and breathing techniques (known as *pranayama*). But this type of yoga—*hatha* yoga—is simply one route toward the ultimate aim of yoga, which is to feel so profoundly at peace within that we become aware of a connection with everything else in the universe. In India, where yoga originated many thousands of years ago, people follow other yoga paths to the same end-state of harmonious union:

> ## >> **weaving yoga** into your life
>
> - **Try to joyfully accept** your current physical limitations. Learn to work with stiff hamstrings or tight shoulders, rather than struggle against them, and you'll become more adept more quickly.
>
> - **Don't be dispirited** when you first begin yoga. Keep a sense of humor, and be kind to your body, and the knots in your mind will also start to unwind.
>
> - **Be patient and watch your breath** rather than pushing yourself to compete, and soon you will experience the bliss of yoga.

bhakti yoga, the path of religious worship; *karma* yoga, doing selfless service for others (Mother Teresa epitomizes this path of yoga); *jnana* yoga, studying yogic philosophy; and *raja* yoga, meditation. Each of these yoga paths suits a different personality type. You have probably turned to *hatha* yoga, the physical aspect of yoga, because, like many of us in the West, you are interested in boosting your health and well-being, and would like to achieve a little more inner peace. As you clean and loosen out your body with its postures, you taste the lightness of being that is *hatha* yoga.

Finding a teacher

When you practice yoga with a teacher, you gain expert advice, as well as invaluable hands-on adjustments. Working with a teacher also helps you gain the confidence to progress to more difficult poses and to work with breathing and meditation techniques. If you attend a regular yoga class, you will also build up a network of supportive fellow students to help you maintain motivation.

But how do you find a teacher to suit you, and a style of yoga from the many confusing options on offer? The best way is to visit a yoga center or gym close to your home or workplace. You can also look for local classes on notice boards in your doctors' office and library, for example. Ask for a list of classes and a description of the style of class if it is not a general "hatha yoga" class (which may draw on a mix of styles—hatha yoga can be taught in myriad ways). Iyengar yoga, the most practiced form of yoga across the globe, focuses on alignment and precision in the physical postures using props such as blocks and belts, and offers a sound foundation for beginners. If you enjoy fast-moving exercise, you might try Ashtanga vinyasa classes, which teach a seamless flow of postures (classes might be called vinyasa flow, dynamic, or power yoga). If you prefer a more esoteric approach that includes chanting and a focus on breathing, meditation, and energy-raising techniques, look out for Sivananda or Kundalini yoga. If you have an ongoing health problem, try therapeutic Iyengar yoga or Viniyoga, which tailors sequences of poses to suit your particular healing needs. If you are pregnant or postpartum, find a class especially geared for you. What's important is that you find the teacher inspiring and approachable. In the end this matters more than the type of yoga you follow.

A teacher offers hands-on adjustments while you hold a pose, which help you to relax effortlessly into the posture and to let go of held-in tension.

>> **advice** for beginners

Once you are on your mat, following the sequences set out in this book, you'll find the 15 minutes fly by as you focus on getting to know your body and mind better. What is more tricky is maintaining the enthusiasm and motivation to roll out the mat in the first place. These tips may help.

The most important advice a teacher can offer beginners to yoga is to make the time to roll out their mats. Practicing in the same place and at the same time can help maintain motivation. Decide on a time and write it into your daybook, thinking of it as an appointment you cannot miss. Indeed, this may be one of the most important appointments you make during a day since it allows you to devote time to looking after yourself. This not only makes you feel great, it sets you up for success in every other part of your day, whether that includes achieving work tasks or mixing with other people.

Setting practice times

Early morning is traditionally considered the best time of day to practice yoga. Try setting your alarm 30 minutes earlier than usual. Take a shower and then practice in the quiet period before the rest of your household awakes. It is interesting to note how this period of reflection first thing can make your home life feel less stressed.

Late afternoon or early evening make good alternative practice times, especially if you need an energy boost or would like to wind down after a hectic day. Wash before you begin and make sure your stomach is empty: let two hours pass after a meal before you practice.

Planning the session

At the start of any yoga session, spend a few minutes sitting, or lying on your back with your knees bent and feet flat on the floor. Close your

>> **before** you begin

- **Remove your watch**, glasses, and any jewelery that might get in the way of your practice. If you have long hair, tie it back.

- **Gather together your props**, which may include a belt and yoga blocks, a chair or bolsters, plus a blanket to keep you warm in the final relaxation pose.

- **Turn off your phone**, and any other sensory distractions, such as the radio or music.

- **Close the door** and make sure those who share your home know not to disturb you.

eyes and look inside yourself, watching your breath flow in and out completely naturally. Then carefully follow the warm-up exercises before beginning the postures. Allow at least five minutes after finishing the routine to lie in the final relaxation pose that ends all yoga sessions.

Take it slowly

Yoga is all about getting to know your capabilities and limitations—but you have the rest of your life to complete this study. Do not feel pressured to push it too far or too fast in the early weeks and months, and do let go of any thoughts of perfection. Yoga is not competitive.

Follow your breath

Tune into your breath not only at the beginning of each session, but in every posture to see what it tells you about your practice. If your breathing becomes ragged or uneven at any time take it as a sign to ease off a little. When you arrive in a pose, explore whether breathing out any tension makes you feel more comfortable, and whether the in-breath allows you to expand and reach a little farther. With time, breath-awareness will become second nature.

Listen to your body

Honor the messages your body sends. If your knees or lower back hurt, for example, take it as an instruction to refer to the easier version of the posture. Acknowledge your limitations, taking things slowly and not progressing to the stronger stretches in the sequences until fully ready—but do not accept your current limitations as your fate. Yoga encourages us to explore the boundaries of what we can do, and to challenge ourselves, but without pursuing perfection, which may lead to physical injury and to unhelpful emotions such as anger or pride. The key to a fulfilling yoga practice is to let expectations go, but to keep pushing into your "edges." Try to incorporate some yoga poses into your everyday life, for example, practice leg raises while you are on the phone or sit on the floor with your back straight while you are reading or watching television, instead of slouching on the sofa, and you will soon notice a real difference.

Incorporate yoga into your daily activities. Sitting on the floor with your legs stretched out in front of you and a straight back will help improve your posture and aid you in your yoga practice.

>> **practicing** safely

Yoga is about knowing yourself. It is important not to push your body beyond its limits. If some of the postures are difficult to start with, feel pleased that you have a challenge ahead of you. For more difficult poses, there are easier options throughout the book for you to refer to.

If you are not used to doing exercise, it is important that you learn the difference between sweet pain—a good, stretchy feeling in the muscles—and sour, or negative, pain—a sharp or nagging pain. This can take time to understand; go slowly. To begin with, you may feel some stiffness for a day or two afterward, but this will soon pass. Do not force your body into positions that it cannot perform. If you find that a pose creates negative pain or tension in a part of your body, ease off. Always veer to the safe side and modify the pose, referring to the easier option, or use equipment (shown on pp16–17) to help you in positions that cause you difficulty.

Always practice yoga on an empty stomach. Allow two to three hours to elapse after a meal before starting yoga.

If you have a specific injury, are pregnant, or have any other health concerns, consult a doctor before using this book. If you feel dizzy, experience chest pain or heart irregularity, or become short of breath while practicing yoga, stop immediately.

Use your environment to help you. Use a shelf for support for a modified standing bend instead of Downward Dog (p25) and a wall or door to lean your legs up against at the end of a tiring day.

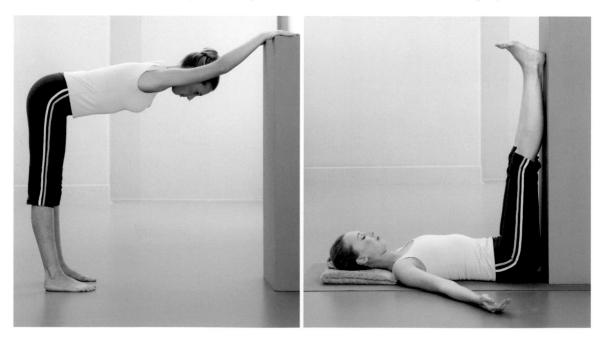

>> **before** you begin

- **Consult** a doctor before practicing yoga if you have an injury, any health concerns, or you are pregnant.

- **Practice** on an empty stomach. Allow three hours to pass after a large meal, two hours after a light meal, and one hour after a snack.

- **Do not overreach** yourself. Take it slowly at first and stop if you are experiencing any negative pain or tension.

- **Refer to the easier options** where relevant and use props to help you in difficult poses.

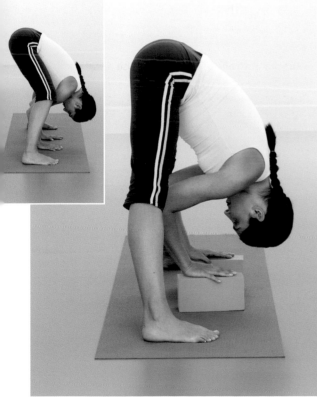

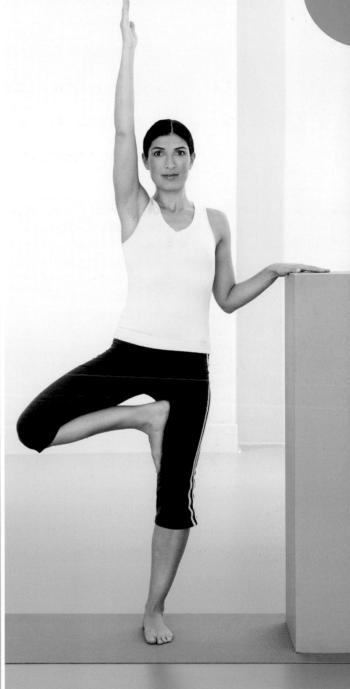

If you find it difficult to reach the floor in a standing forward bend, bend your knees (see inset) or place a block under your hands.

Balancing can be hard at first for beginners or if you are feeling particularly tired. Use a wall to lean against or a surface to hold on to.

>> **clothing** and equipment

There is no need to spend vast amounts of money on specific equipment or clothes. Invest in a yoga mat, but just wear comfortable clothing, and if you need props to help you with the more difficult poses, use household items that have the same effect as the yoga equipment available to buy.

When you are new to yoga, you may find that you need all the help you can get to discipline yourself. It helps if you find a little spot in your home that you can practice in regularly and where you will not be disturbed. Tell the people you share your home with that you want at least 15 minutes of private time. Make sure that the phone is silenced and that you are away from your computer and daily chores. If you use the same place each time for your practice, you may find that it develops a special energy that you associate with your practice. You may feel you want to light a candle, place a bowl of flowers there, or a picture of someone who inspires you.

Practice in a quiet, clean, warm environment. A wooden floor is ideal, or one that allows you to practice without a mat. However, if the surface of the floor is slippery, you must use a yoga mat. As a beginner, you may want to be close to a wall when practicing, to help support you when balancing.

Clothing

Before starting, change into comfortable clothes that do not restrict you in any way. You may also feel you want to wash before you practice. The clothing you wear must be comfortable and flexible, with elastic waist bands. Fabrics that are made from natural fibers work well, since they help the body to breathe. Wear shorts, leggings, cropped pants, or pants that you can roll up, which allow you to see if your legs and feet are correctly aligned. Bare feet are essential so that you are able to stretch out and invigorate your feet.

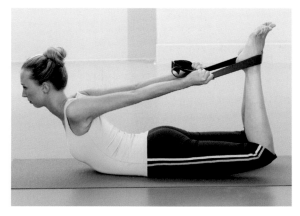

Wrapping a belt around your feet can help you hold a pose that you otherwise may not be able to (see Full Bow, page 79).

Equipment

If your floor is slippery you will need to buy a yoga mat, but for the other equipment, use general household items that have the same effect. As you become more experienced, you may find that you want to buy equipment specially designed for yoga (see resources, pp124–125 for retailers).

● **Using a belt** helps to deepen a pose without applying force and to hold a pose in correct alignment. You may also need to use one for poses where you are unable to reach your hands together (see Cow Face Pose, p71) or to help bring your legs off the floor (see Full Bow, p79). You can use a bathrobe belt at first.

mat

- **Blocks** are useful if your hands cannot quite reach the floor, or if you need more height under your sitting bones. Sitting on them also helps keep you straight. Different-sized blocks are available to buy, but you can use telephone books or other books instead. Cover them or tape them up so that they are firmer.

- **Placing a bolster** underneath you when lying flat helps open up your chest. You can also use it to sit on or place it under your knees to relax your back in the final relaxation (see p120).

- **Lightweight blankets or towels** are useful to have on hand. These can be folded or rolled up neatly to support you and make you more comfortable when sitting or lying. You can also use them to cover you to keep you warm during relaxation. Place an eye pad over your eyes during the final relaxation.

- **Place a chair or stool** near to you when you are practicing. If you feel particularly stiff and it is difficult for you to take your hands to the floor, use

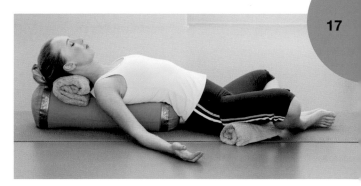

Use a bolster and towels to make you more comfortable. Lying on a bolster also helps open your chest, helping you breathe.

a chair to put your hands on to help you bend over. Use a chair or stool for resting your calves during the final relaxation and also for support when it is hard to balance in the standing poses.

Classic yoga equipment is available from specific yoga stores and online. At first, use household items to help you feel more comfortable and relaxed and to modify the more difficult poses.

blanket

block

towel

belt

cushion

eye pad

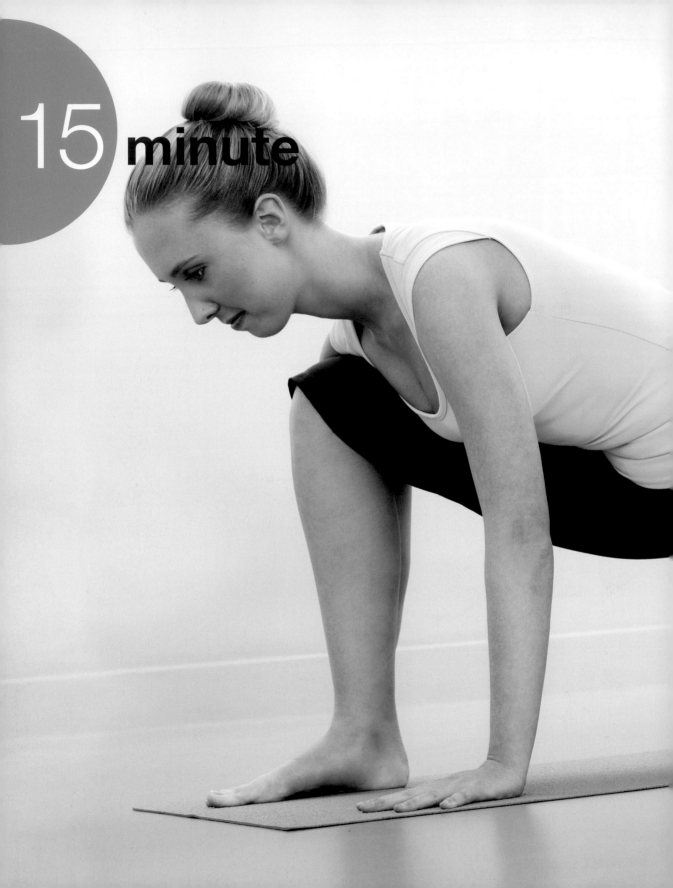

15 minute

rise and shine >>

Start the morning
with a series of gentle,
flowing movements
to prepare you for
the day ahead

>> **rise** and shine

Getting up in the morning can be hard. This sequence is designed to help you get rid of stiffness, focus, and become energized for the day ahead. Performing the Sun Salutation gently oils and loosens the joints and elasticates the spine.

Spend just a few minutes every day, lying on your back with your knees bent toward your body and your feet flat on the floor, just listening to your breath. It is amazing how much more aware you become of your body. Place a block or folded blanket under your head to make you more comfortable. Do not try to change the breath, just listen to it and notice how it becomes more even and quiets the mind. Observing the breath throughout all of the sequences is very important and stops you from going too far in your practice. If the breath becomes uneven and jagged, you are pushing yourself too far in the posture.

The exercises

The warm-up loosens you up in preparation for the Sun Salutation. If you are short of time in the morning, perform the warm-up on its own, as a quick way to get you started with your day.

The Sun Salutation is a series of gentle, flowing movements that are synchronized with the breath. There are many variations; this is just one example. Each position counteracts the one before, stretching the body in a different way and alternately expanding and contracting the chest to regulate the breathing. It helps the body gain flexibility. It regulates the breath and focuses the mind and it is believed to reduce lethargy and combat depression.

When you first begin, you may feel very clumsy. Take it slowly and refer to the easier options, for example, bring your foot forward with your hand

> ### >> **tips for** rise and shine
>
> - **Learn to watch the breath** by lying quietly and listening to your natural breath coming and going.
>
> - **Do not push yourself too far.** If your breath becomes rough or irregular, back off a little.
>
> - **Do not worry** if your breath does not flow smoothly initially during the Sun Salutation. Take as many breaths as you need.
>
> - **Be patient** and keep a sense of humor. There are easier options for you to perform where poses are particularly difficult.

into a lunge, if you are very stiff (see p30). Do not worry if your breath does not flow easily at first, take extra breaths whenever necessary. With practice, you will begin to flow into each movement with one breath. Over time, increase the number of rounds from two to however many you feel comfortable with, making sure you perform an even number. Be patient, keep a sense of humor, and practice, practice, practice.

Be patient and take it slowly at first. If you are unable to perform the more difficult Cobra pose (right), practice the Sphinx (p30) until you feel ready to move on to the Cobra.

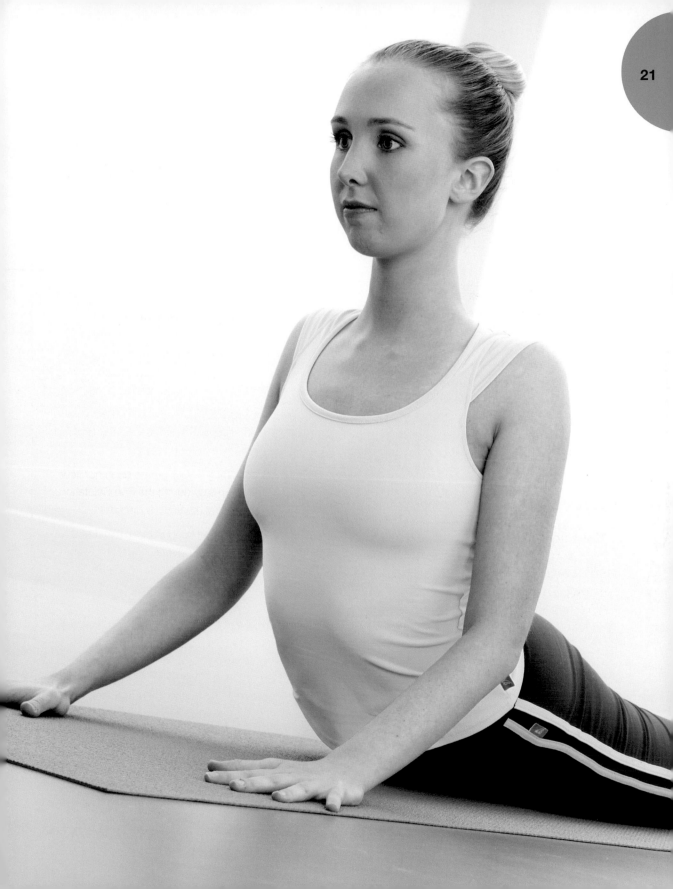

>> **rise & shine** listening to your breath

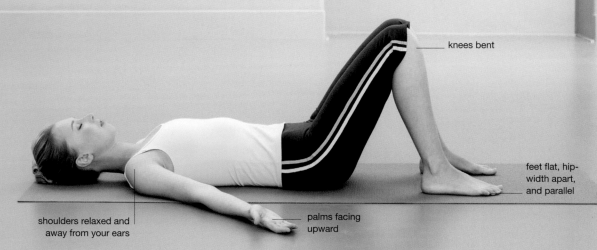

1 Lie flat on your back with your knees bent and your arms out at 45 degrees to your body. Keep the back of your neck long. Close your eyes and listen to your natural breath coming and going. To bring more awareness into your lungs, breathe in steadily for 3 counts and out for 4, repeating several times.

knees bent

feet flat, hip-width apart, and parallel

shoulders relaxed and away from your ears

palms facing upward

2 Inhale and bend your knees toward your chest, with your hands resting on your knees. Keep the back of your neck long.

knees bent towards your body

keep your neck long

3 Exhale and stretch your right leg out along the floor, keeping your leg straight and strong. Flex your foot and keep it about 1 in (2.5 cm) off the floor. Inhale and bend both knees toward your chest. Exhale and repeat with your left leg. Repeat for both legs once more, returning both knees back toward your body (see Step 2).

stretch along the inside of your leg to the inner heel

foot flexed and 1 in (2.5 cm) off the floor

4 Keep your knees bent toward your chest and stretch your arms out to your sides. Exhale and take both knees down toward your right elbow. At the same time, turn your head and abdomen toward the left. Inhale and come back to the center (see inset). Exhale and repeat on your left side, as you turn your head and navel toward the right. Repeat on both sides, returning to the center each time.

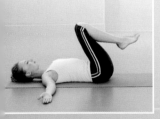

head and abdomen turned away from your knees

arms out to the side at shoulder-height

palms facing upward

knee and foot on the floor, if they will go

>> **rise & shine** rock and roll/circling

5 Start to awaken the spine. With your knees still hugged toward your body, but holding the back of your knees, gently rock backward and forward on your spine. Inhale as you roll back. Exhale as you roll forward. Repeat several times. If your back feels too stiff, just roll gently from side to side instead.

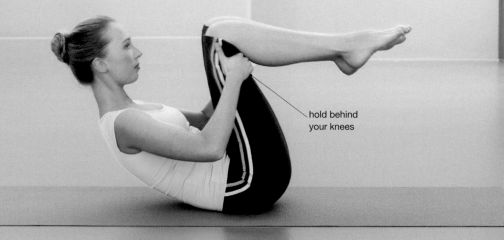

hold behind
your knees

6 Turn to the side to come onto all-fours, facing the front of the mat. Your hands shoulder-width apart, facing forward, and your knees are hip-width apart with the tops of your feet flat on the floor. Circle your hips 3 times to the left, taking one full breath for each circle. Feel like you are drawing a circle with your navel out to your hips. Repeat to the right. Feel your lower back relaxing.

tops of feet on
the floor

hands shoulder-width
apart and facing
forward

7 Inhale and look ahead. Keep your shoulders away from your ears and your tailbone back. Exhale, rounding your back and looking to your navel, as you stretch your buttocks back and down toward your heels, with your head resting on the floor for **Child's Pose**. Your hands are on the floor in front of you. At first, your head may not touch the floor and your buttocks may not reach your heels. If your knees feel very stiff, place a blanket behind the knees. If your ankles hurt, place a rolled towel under them.

buttocks stretching down toward your heels

point fingers forward

easier option

push sitbones up

8 Inhale and come up onto all-fours again, placing your feet flat on the floor. Look ahead. Keep your shoulders away from your ears and draw your navel back to the spine. Exhale and tuck your toes under, as you come up into **Downward Dog**. Push away and down with your heels and up with your buttocks, lengthening your spine. Bend your knees if your hamstrings feel too tight (see inset). Repeat Steps 7–8 once more.

neck relaxed

push heels away and down

straight arms

9 Gently walk your feet and hands toward each other until you are in a **Standing Forward Bend**. Your feet are parallel and hip-width apart. If your back feels stiff, keep your legs bent (see inset). Inhale, bending your knees more. Exhale, lifting your kneecaps and sucking the front of your thighs up and back. Feel your feet growing roots down into the floor, relaxed, but grounding down. Breathe freely.

easier option

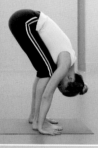

feet parallel and hip-width apart

arms reaching up

10 Inhale and sweep your arms out to the side and up over your head as you come up to standing for **Extended Mountain Pose**. By the time your arms are over your head, your legs are straight. Stretch all along the outside of your body to your finger tips.

feet pushing down

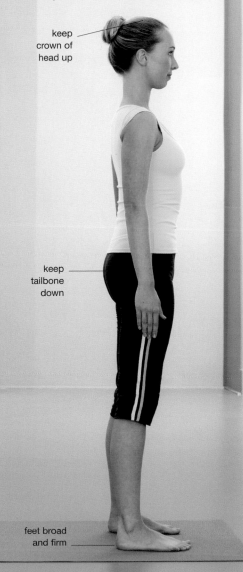

11 Exhale, bringing your arms out and down by your side. Step your feet together at the front of the mat and stand in **Mountain Pose**. Feel a plumb line through the center of your body. Get ready for 2 rounds of **Sun Salutation**.

keep crown of head up

keep tailbone down

feet broad and firm

12 Exhale and bring your hands into **Prayer Position** in front of your chest. Inhale and sweep your arms out and up over your head (see inset). Look up.

prayer position

>> **rise & shine** sun salutation

13 Exhale and swing your arms out and down as you bend forward into **Standing Forward Bend**. Place your hands on the floor by the side of your feet, but allow your knees to bend if necessary. Keep your head relaxed.

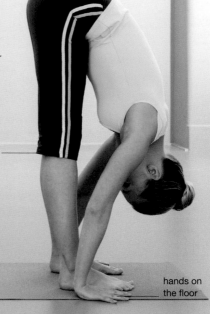

bend knees if
need be

hands on
the floor

14 Inhale and bring your right leg back and your knee to the floor. Place your hands on the floor on either side of your front foot for a **Lunge**.

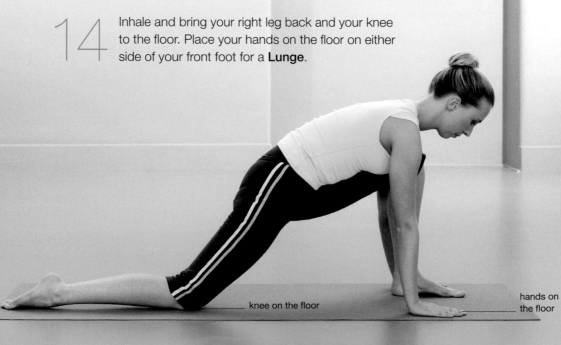

knee on the floor

hands on
the floor

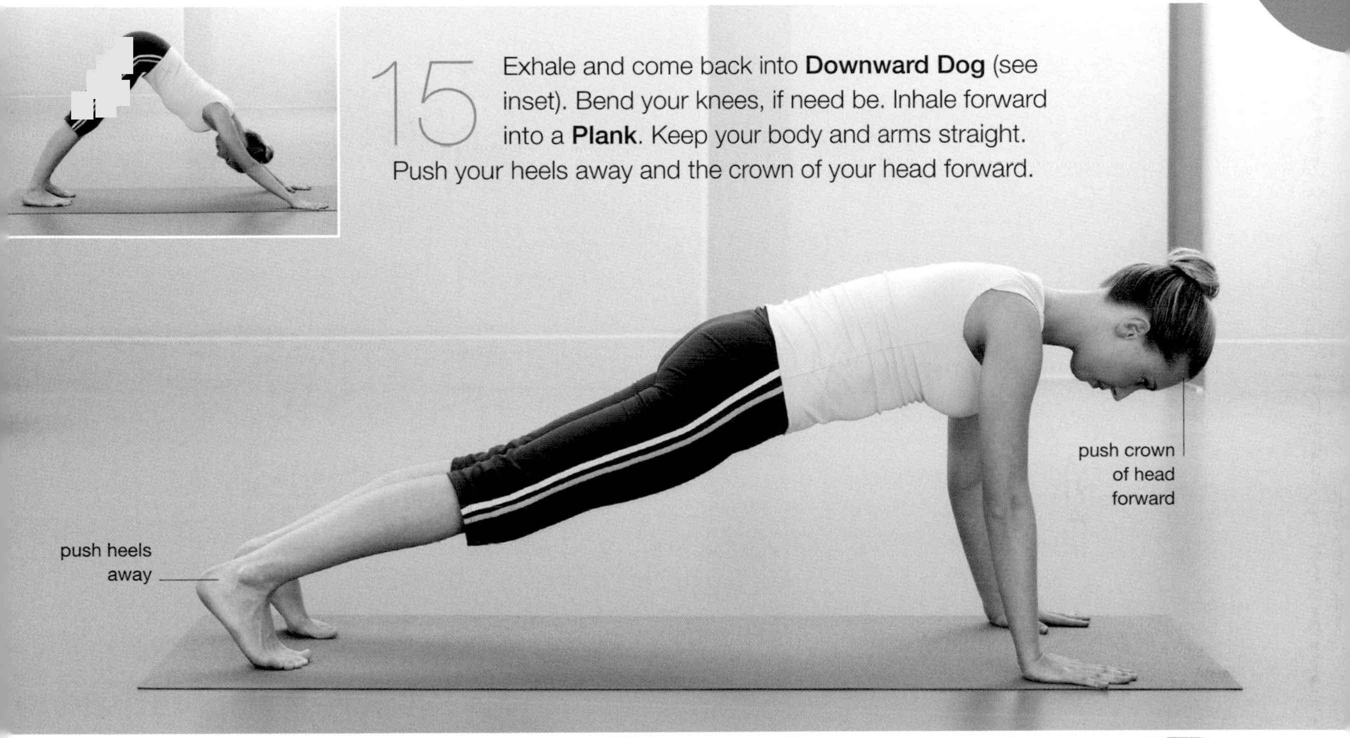

15 Exhale and come back into **Downward Dog** (see inset). Bend your knees, if need be. Inhale forward into a **Plank**. Keep your body and arms straight. Push your heels away and the crown of your head forward.

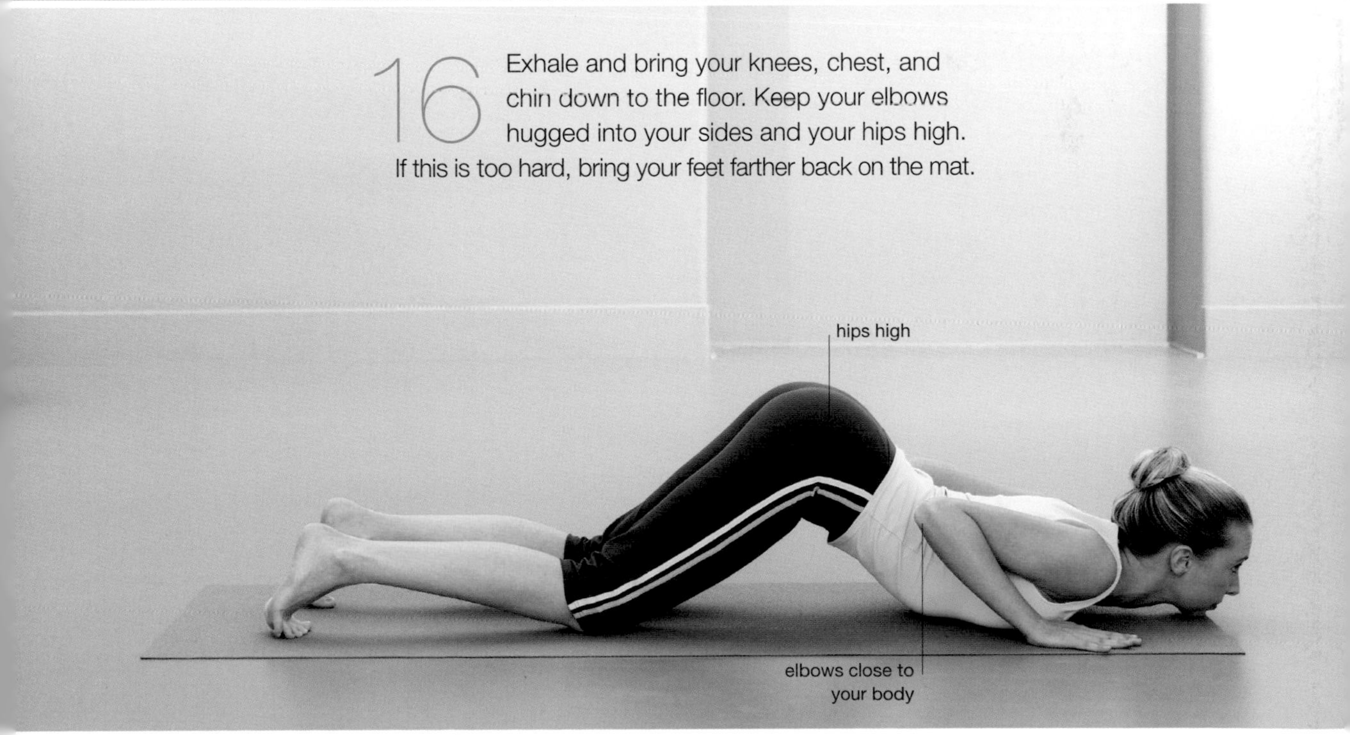

push crown
of head
forward

push heels
away

16 Exhale and bring your knees, chest, and chin down to the floor. Keep your elbows hugged into your sides and your hips high. If this is too hard, bring your feet farther back on the mat.

hips high

elbows close to
your body

17 Inhale into the **Cobra**. Keep your elbows hugged into your sides and bring the tops of your feet and legs down onto the floor. Lengthen all along your legs to the inner heel. Push down with your pubic bone and lift your navel to your chest. Keep your shoulders down, away from your ears. Lift upward with the top of your chest. Look ahead. If this is difficult, place your elbows and forearms on the floor in front of you for the **Sphinx** (see inset).

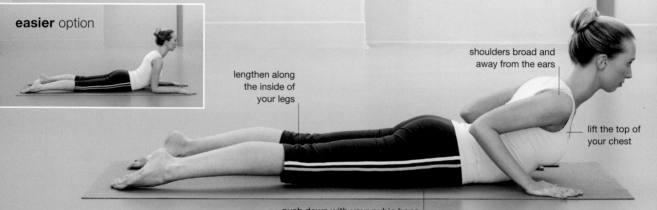

easier option

shoulders broad and away from the ears

lengthen along the inside of your legs

lift the top of your chest

push down with your pubic bone

18 Exhale and tuck your toes under and push up into the **Downward Dog**. Take a couple of breaths here. Inhale and bring your right foot forward, in between your hands, as you bring your left knee to the floor (see inset). Look ahead. If this is difficult, use your hand to bring the foot forward (see easier option).

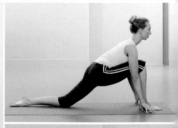

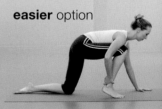

push up as high as possible

easier option

push mat back with balls of feet

push mat forward with hands

19 Exhale and bring your back foot forward to join your front foot. Place your hands on the floor on either side of your feet for a **Standing Forward Bend**, keeping your knees bent if necessary. Keep your heels firm on the floor, but bring your weight farther forward, so that you can feel your front thigh muscles lifting, the backs of your knees opening, and your calves stretching down to your heels.

20 Sweep your arms out to the side and up over your head as you come back up to standing. Look up. Exhale and bring your hands down the center line to the chest into prayer position (see inset). Look ahead. Repeat Steps 12–20 on your left side to complete one full round of the **Sun Salutation**, and then repeat another full round. Bring your hands down by the side of your body for **Mountain Pose**. Listen to your breath coming and going. Step back to the middle of the mat.

heels firm on floor

21 Kneel down to **Child's Pose**. Allow your big toes to touch, but keep your heels apart. Rest your forehead on the floor and let your sitting bones sink down to your heels. Bring your arms by your feet, palms facing upward. Breathe naturally. As you inhale, you may feel your breath moving in your lower back. Exhale and relax.

toes touching and heels apart

forehead rests on the floor

22 Roll up, vertebra by vertebra, with your head coming up last, until you are sitting up straight for the **Lion**. Place your hands on your knees. If it is uncomfortable to kneel, place a cushion behind your knees and a rolled towel under your ankles. Inhale. Open your mouth wide and stretch your tongue out; look in between your eyebrows and exhale through your mouth with a roar (a "ha" sound). Inhale and close your eyes and mouth. Repeat twice more.

straight arms

23 Move your hands farther back up your thighs with your palms facing upward. Close your eyes. Breathe in as if you are smelling a beautiful flower. Exhale and let go. Sit quietly, focusing on your breath coming and going.

palms facing
upward

24 Lie on your back with your knees bent and your feet flat on the floor (hip-width apart and parallel). Lift your head and look down your center line to see that you are straight. Place your head on the floor and your arms away from your body. Lengthen one leg out along the floor and then the other, ready for the final relaxation. Stay here for 2–5 minutes. Place a folded blanket under your head, a cushion under your knees and an eye pad on your eyes, if you wish, to make you more comfortable.

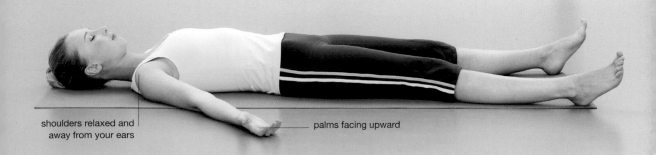

shoulders relaxed and
away from your ears

palms facing upward

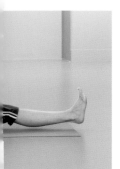

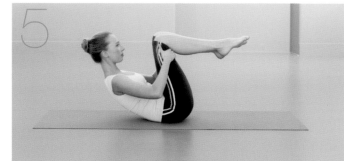

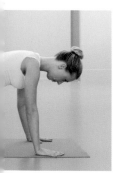

▲ **Rock and Roll**, page 24

ss, page 23

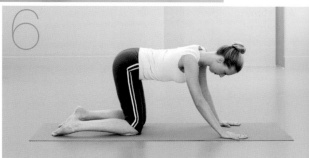

▲ **Circling**, page 24

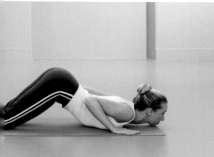

▲ **Cobra**, page 30

I chin to floor, page 29

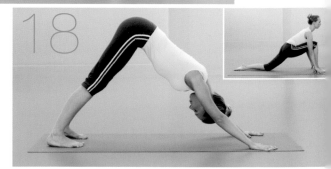

▲ **Downward Dog/Lunge**, page 30

rise and shine at a glance

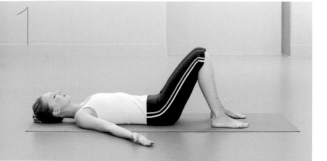

▲ **Listening to your breath**, page 22

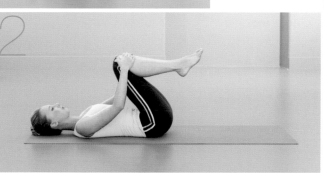

▲ **Listening to your breath**, easing out stiffness, page 22

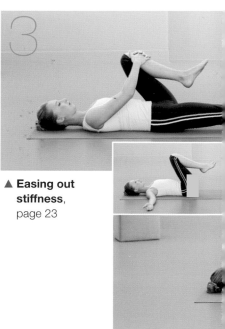

▲ **Easing out stiffness**, page 23

▲ **Easing out stiffne**

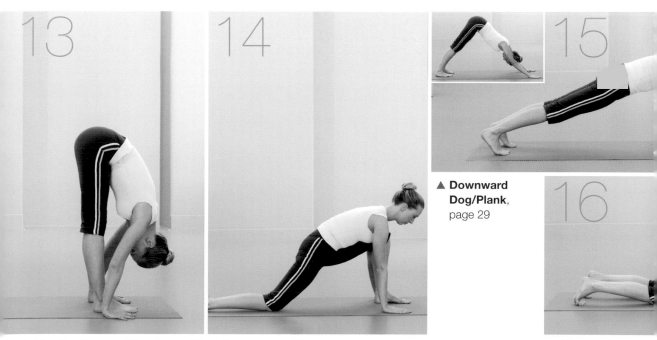

▲ **Standing Forward Bend**, page 28   ▲ **Lunge**, page 28

▲ **Downward Dog/Plank**, page 29

▲ **Knees, chest, an**

rise and shine >>

15 minute **summary**

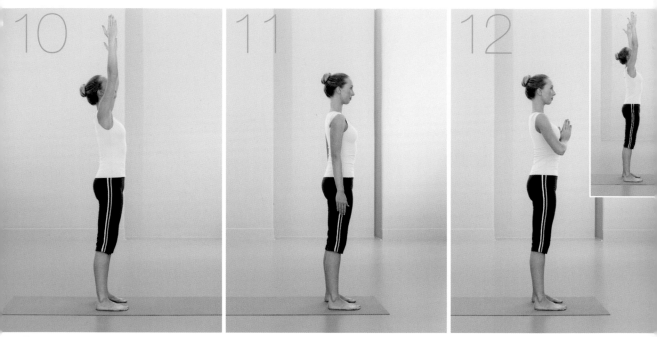

▲ **Extended Mountain Pose**, page 26 ▲ **Ready for Sun Salutation**, page 27 ▲ **Prayer Position**, page 27

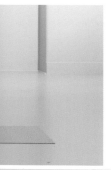

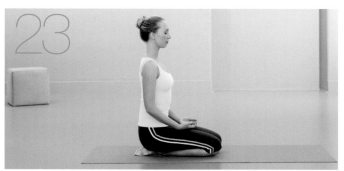

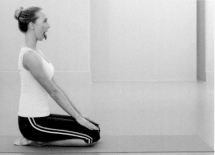

▲ **Final Relaxation**, watching breath, page 33

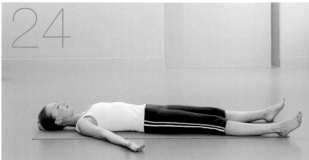

▲ **Final Relaxation**, page 33

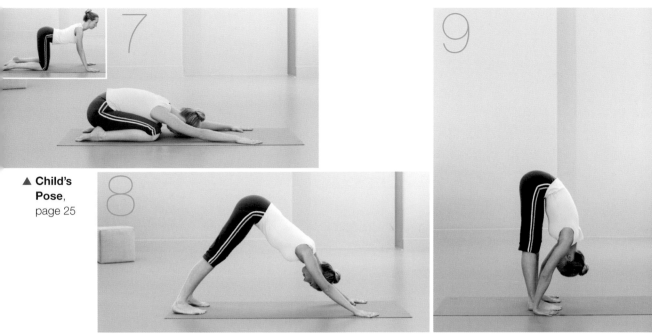

▲ **Child's Pose**, page 25

▲ **Downward Dog**, page 25

▲ **Standing Forward Bend**, page 26

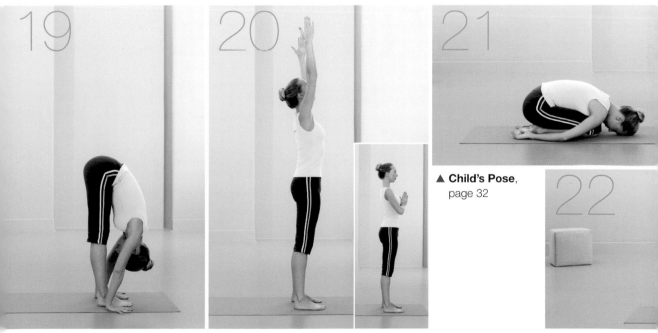

▲ **Standing Forward Bend**, page 31 ▲ **Sun Salutation** ends, page 31. Repeat 12–20

▲ **Child's Pose**, page 32

▲ **Lion**, page 32

>> **rise and shine** FAQs

Yoga is not a competitive sport and it takes patience. Do not feel disheartened if the poses do not come easily to you at first. Here are some tips to help you with form and getting your breathing right. Heed this advice, make time to practice, and soon you will be reaping the benefits.

>> ### I'm finding it hard to find time to practice. Any advice?

People often say this to me but if you think about it, it is not usually time, but personal discipline that we are lacking. We have the discipline to go to work and care for our families, but frequently, we don't have the discipline care for after ourselves. Treat your exercise as something you just do every day, like brushing your teeth. If you spend 15 minutes a day on yourself, you will find that you will have more energy and become more efficient, so in fact, you will have more time.

>> ### Why should I practice yoga in the morning? I'm very stiff when I wake up and don't feel like it.

This is precisely why you should practice yoga! It is very common to feel stiff in the early morning. First, think about the way you sleep and try not to sleep on your front. Steps 1–8 in this sequence, as well as steps 3, 10, and 11 in Strengthening and 2–4 in Winding Down, will help ease your stiffness. If you practice for 15 minutes every day for one month, you should see results. Many people prefer to practice in the morning when it is quieter and there are fewer distractions.

>> ### What do you mean by "watching your breath"?

When you first begin yoga it is very easy for your mind to be elsewhere. Use your breath as a focus point. Be aware of each inhale and each exhale. Don't try to force or change anything. The inhalation takes you to the parts of the body that need attention. The exhalation is when you do the work in the posture. You then lengthen on the inhalation. As you become more familiar with the breath patterns, your breathing will become smoother and freer.

>> I can't touch my toes in the Standing Forward Bend. It's impossible. Help!

Initially, if you're very stiff, place your hands on a table or other surface and walk your feet away until your legs and arms form a right angle (see bottom left picture on page 14). Feel a stretch in your shoulders and armpits and make sure your legs are straight. If you are not far off from reaching the floor, bend your knees slightly or place your hands on a block.

>> My lower back hurts in the Cobra. Can you help?

Never continue with a pose if it causes you negative pain. Do not come up so far with your chest. Lengthen your tailbone toward your heels and push your pubic bone down into the floor. Make your legs feel stronger by pushing your feet down into the floor. If the Cobra is too difficult, practice the Sphinx (p30).

>> My feet and knees hurt in the kneeling exercises. What should I do?

If your feet hurt when you kneel, roll a towel, and place it under your ankles, or fold a couple of blankets and stack them on top of each other. Kneel on the blankets with your feet hanging off the back. Over time, the tops of your feet will stretch out and you will be able to reduce the height. A good, healthy stretch on the tops of your feet is positive pain. Knees have to be taken care of and treated with great respect because they often take the strain when other parts of our body are not supporting us correctly. A stretch in your front thigh is positive, but if your knees hurt when kneeling, place a folded blanket behind your knees and a block under your buttocks until you can sit straight and relatively comfortably.

>> How do I benefit from the Lion?

The Lion pose exercises facial muscles and relaxes the tongue, an exercise they rarely get in the course of our everyday lives, and is particulary beneficial to people who experience tension in the jaw. With regular practice, it is believed to make speech clearer and is recommended for stammerers. It may also help alleviate bad breath and clean the tongue. Try to touch your chin with your tongue for a good stretch. On each roar, focus your eyes on a different spot: between your eyebrows, the tip of your nose, and a spot far ahead.

15 minute

strengthening
the body >>

Root into the ground and
engage your core muscles
to build up inner strength
and improve posture

>> **strengthening**

If you get tired standing, feel lethargic, or have a stiff neck or rounded shoulders, you will benefit from the inner strength this sequence promotes. It also counteracts a tendency to slump and breathe shallowly, and helps you distribute your weight evenly throughout your body.

For a moment, try out what it feels like to stand well. Place your feet hip-width apart and send your body weight equally down both legs and feet. Visualize the front and back of your heart opening and your head moving up and back. Breathe through your nose, feeling the breath caress your throat. How do you feel? Tall, light, powerful, and full of zest? This is the energizing transformation yoga can bring to your life if you follow the 15-minute sequence that follows, which teaches how it feels to be strong and well supported within.

Inner strength comes from rooting into the ground with your feet and drawing the power this generates up through your body's central axis, so that your upper body feels supported and able to relax. You gain the sense of a plumb line dropping from the top of the back of the skull down the spine to the sitting bones, which restores a natural, healthy posture.

The exercises

The warm-ups and breathing exercise put you in touch with the core muscles around your navel that support your lower back. As you practice, focus on drawing your abdominal muscles toward your spine without tensing your stomach. At the same time draw up your pelvic floor for extra support.

This refreshing sequence contains plenty of movements to strengthen your legs, and by promoting circulation and increasing mobility, it also relieves body tension. The Tiptoes pose cultivates balance while engaging the calves and thighs, and

> ## >> **tips for** strengthening
>
> - **Engage your core muscles** as you root down through the feet in standing poses, feeling your pelvic floor naturally lift and your navel draw toward your spine.
>
> - **Watch your knees** in wide-legged standing poses; they should never hurt. Keep each knee in line with the middle of the foot rather than rolling toward the big toe by lifting your thigh muscles and turning them out.
>
> - **Use props** if you feel exhausted or are menstruating, reaching out to a wall or a chair for support in the standing poses.

when the feet ground strongly into the floor, the upper body gains a welcome sense of lightness and relaxation. The Lateral Stretch and Rhythmic Twist bring increased awareness to the spine and shoulders, while the Squat loosens the hips. The Horse tests your leg strength—try to ride out any shakiness—before you tackle yoga's classical standing poses. At the end of the sequence, you will really appreciate the supported relaxation pose.

Standing balances encourage powerful concentration and focus in the mind as well as building strength and mobility in the lower and upper body.

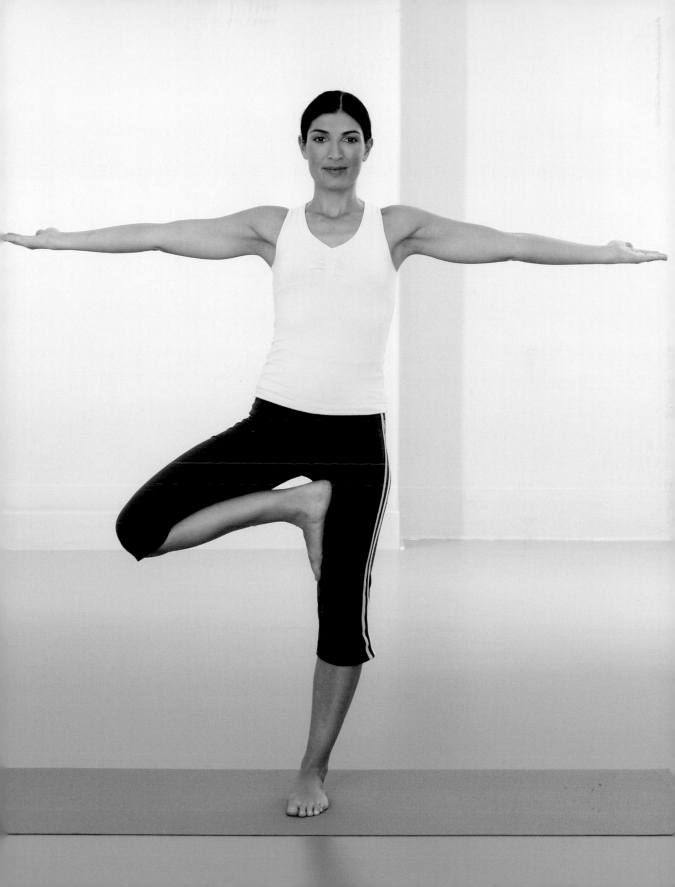

>> **strengthening** quieting the mind

1 Sit cross-legged on a block or cushion with your back straight and your hands resting on your knees or thighs. If it is difficult to sit straight, make your base higher. If your knees don't touch the floor, put cushions under your thighs. Watch your breath and allow your mind to quiet.

shoulders relaxed

elbows slightly bent

palms facing upward

sit on a block or cushion

2 Remain cross-legged for **Shining Skull** (*Kapalabhati*), an exercise to cleanse the lungs and mind. Concentrate on a strong exhalation as you pull your abdomen in and then immediately allow it to relax so that the inhalation (see inset) is spontaneous and relaxed. Repeat 10 pumps quickly. Return to natural inhalation and exhalation for a few breaths before each round. Repeat twice.

contract abdominal muscles quickly on exhalation

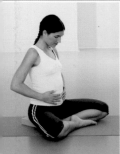

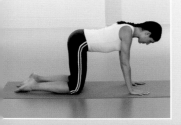

3 Come onto all-fours for a **Diagonal Stretch**. Exhale and stretch your left arm forward and your right leg back. Keep your shoulders away from your ears and your leg straight and strong. Draw your abdomen back to the spine to support your lower back. Inhale and come back to the center. Repeat on your other side and repeat again on both sides.

abdomen is drawing back to the spine

hands are in line with shoulders

knees are in line with hips

4 For a **Plank**, bring your elbows down to the floor, in line with your shoulders. Place your forearms straight out in front of you on the floor. Exhale and lift your knees off the floor, pushing your heels back and away. Your body should be straight. Draw your abdomen back to the spine. Keep your shoulders away from your ears, your neck long and the crown of your head forward. Breathe naturally.

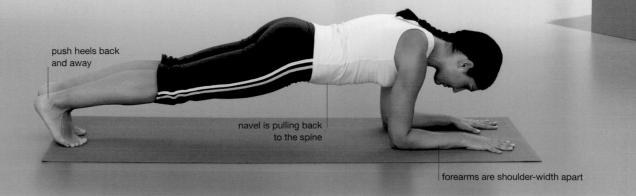

push heels back and away

navel is pulling back to the spine

forearms are shoulder-width apart

>> **strengthening** bent leg dog/forward bend

5 Come back onto all-fours, tucking your toes under. Exhale, lifting your knees off the floor and straightening your legs into **Downward Dog**. Push your sitbones up, relax your head, and keep your arms straight. If your hamstrings feel very tight initially, bend your legs, feeling your spine lengthening. On every exhalation, pull the front of your thighs up to help straighten your legs.

push sitbones up

push the mat forward with your hands

push the mat back with the balls of your feet

6 Walk your hands and feet toward each other into a **Standing Forward Bend**. If your hamstrings feel tight, bend your knees a little (see inset). Over time, as your sitbones shoot up and your feet grow roots down, your legs will gently straighten. If your back hurts at all, bend your knees more or rest your hands on a chair or shelf in a Half Forward Bend (see p14).

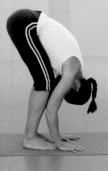

easier option

7 Roll up, vertebra by vertebra, until you are in **Mountain Pose**. Stand with your feet hip-width apart, growing roots down. Draw your abdomen back to the spine. Breathe through your nose, feeling your breath softly caressing the back of your throat.

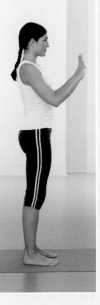

keep crown of head up

draw abdomen back to the spine

keep tailbone down

8 For the **Tiptoes** exercise, bring your hands in front of you at shoulder-height with your palms facing forward and your elbows by your side. Inhale and come up onto the balls of your feet. Exhale and come down. Repeat 4 times.

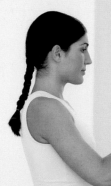

place hands against a wall if balancing is difficult

bring heels up high as you come up onto tiptoes

9 Inhale and move your arms forward and up over your head as you come onto your tiptoes. Stretch up to your fingertips. Exhale, bringing your heels down, and bend your knees into the **Chair Pose**. Inhale, straightening your legs. Exhale, and bring your arms out and down by your side.

arms stay above head for Chair Pose

10 Interlace your fingers for a **Standing Lateral Stretch**. Turn your hands out and push your palms away from you. Inhale, lifting your arms up over your head. Exhale, stretching to the right, with a firm weight on your left foot. Inhale back to the center. Repeat to the left. Change the interlace of your fingers. Repeat once more on both sides.

root down with opposite foot

11 Bring your arms out and down, ready for **Standing Rhythmic Twist**. With your knees slightly bent and your arms hanging loosely by your side, swing your upper body from left to right. Your arms are relaxed and gently swinging from side to side with your hands tapping your body. Breathe naturally as you rhythmically swing.

12 For **Eagle Arms**, lift your arms out to the side and wrap your right arm over your left. Place the fingers of your left hand into your right palm, and bring your thumbs in front of your nose. Push forward with your left hand and pull back with your right.

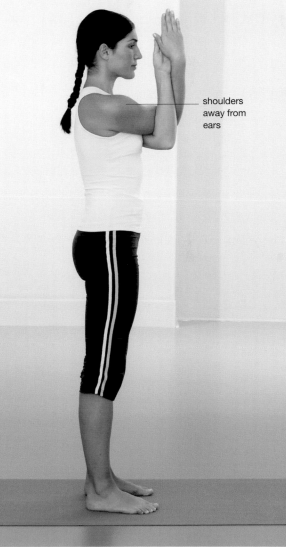

arms relaxed and gently swinging

shoulders away from ears

13 Exhale down into a **Squat**. Feel the weight on the outside of your feet. If it is difficult to squat, just come down as far as you are able, without lifting your heels. Inhale and come back up. Exhale and release your arms out to the side. Switch hands and repeat. Inhale and come up, releasing your arms out and down by your side.

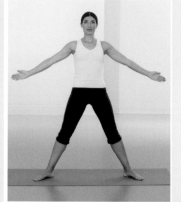

14 Step around to the middle of the mat. Move your feet wide apart and turn them out to 45 degrees. Inhale and bring your arms out and up over your head, palms touching.

knees over feet

tailbone down

feet just wider than hip-width apart

feet wide and turned out at 45 degrees

15 Exhale into the **Horse**, bending your knees so that they are in line with your feet and bringing your hands down through your center line into prayer position. Inhale and push your feet into the floor to straighten your legs. Bring your arms over your head as you come up. Touch your palms together above your head. Repeat once more.

16 Inhale and straighten your legs. Stretch your arms out straight at shoulder height. Turn your right foot out and your left foot in for **Triangle** pose. Exhale out to the right, bringing your right hand to rest on your right shin, and your left arm up, straight. Inhale and look down at your front big toe. Exhale and look ahead. Take a couple of breaths here, come up, and repeat on the left side.

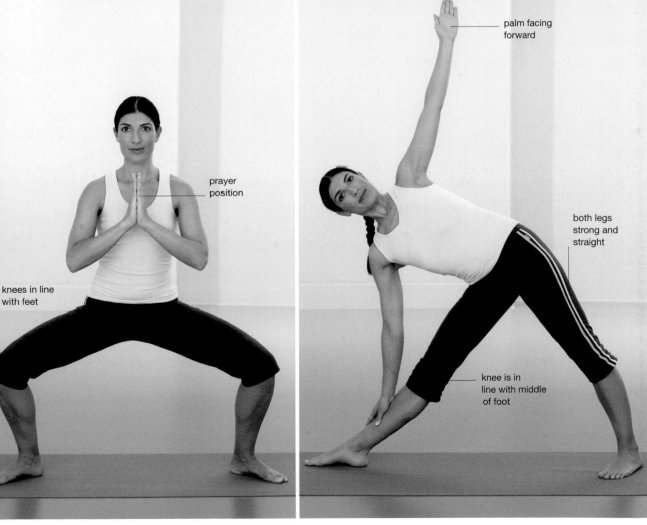

prayer position

knees in line with feet

palm facing forward

both legs strong and straight

knee is in line with middle of foot

17 Inhale and come back up to center. For a **Wide Leg Forward Bend**, rest your hands on your hips. Inhale and look up. Exhale and hinge at your hips, bringing your hands down to the floor. Bend your knees a little, if need be, or use blocks to rest your hands on (see p15, bottom left picture). Walk your feet a little wider apart. Inhale and look ahead. Exhale, let your head go, and bring your hands farther back, in line with your toes (see inset). Inhale and look ahead. Exhale and bring your hands to your hips. Inhale and come up.

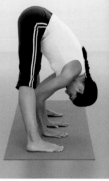

feet parallel

hands in line with shoulders

18 Turn your right foot out and keep your left foot in, ready for **Warrior 2**. Exhale and bend your right knee directly over your ankle. Rotate both your knees away from each other. Keep strong and straight on your left leg all the way to the outside of your foot. Inhale and stretch your arms out, looking out toward your right index finger. Have a couple of breaths here.

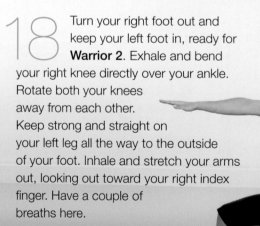

arms out at shoulder height

calf forms a right angle with thigh

rotate knee out

19 For a modified **Side Angle Stretch**, place your right elbow onto your right knee, resting your left hand on the outside of your left thigh. Turn your abdomen and chest up toward the ceiling. Look up at your left shoulder as your right elbow pushes your right knee back and you roll your right buttock under. Feel the stretch through your straight back leg to the outside of your foot. Breathe freely.

leg is straight and strong to the outside of your foot

20 If you want to go further, inhale and stretch your left arm out and up over your head, as you bring your right hand to the floor on the inside of your right foot. Hit your right knee back with your right elbow and roll your right buttock under as you turn your torso upward. Have a couple of breaths here. Inhale and come back up. Repeat Steps 18–20 on your left side.

keep a straight line from your left foot to your fingertips

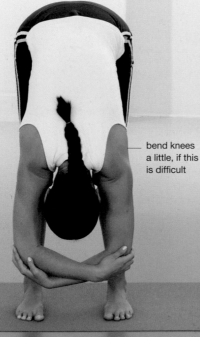

21 Inhale and come back up, bringing your arms down by your side. Stand with your feet hip-width apart, in **Mountain Pose**. With your hands on your hips, hinge forward into a **Standing Forward Bend**. Hold your elbows and release forward. Take a couple of breaths. Inhale and look ahead. Exhale and place your hands on your hips. Inhale and come up with a flat back to **Mountain Pose** with your arms by your side.

22 Step your feet together for **Tree Pose.** Place the sole of your right foot on your inner left thigh. Move your hands into prayer position. If you want to go further, inhale and take your arms over your head (see inset). Bring your arms down through the center line to prayer position. Release your right foot. Bring your feet together and repeat on the other side. If it is difficult to balance, stand next to a wall.

bend knees a little, if this is difficult

press your foot into your thigh and your thigh into your foot

23 Take your chair or stool and place it at the end of the mat. Lie down in front of the chair or stool, with your knees bent toward your chest for a **Back Release** exercise. Hold your knees with your hands. Exhale and hug your knees toward your chest. Inhale and release. Repeat a couple of times.

knees hugged toward chest

24 For the **Final Relaxation**, bring your arms down by your side and rest your calves on the chair or stool. Check that you are straight and close your eyes. Place a blanket under your head if it is more comfortable, and an eye pad on your eyes. Stay here for 2–5 minutes.

neck is long

shoulders relaxed, away from the ears

palms facing upward

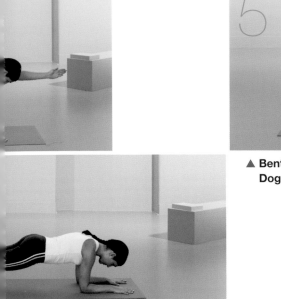

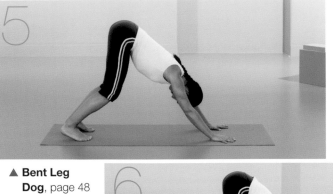

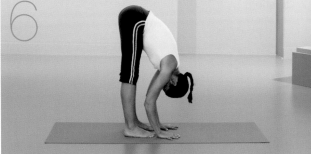

▲ **Bent Leg Dog**, page 48

▲ **Standing Forward Bend**, page 48

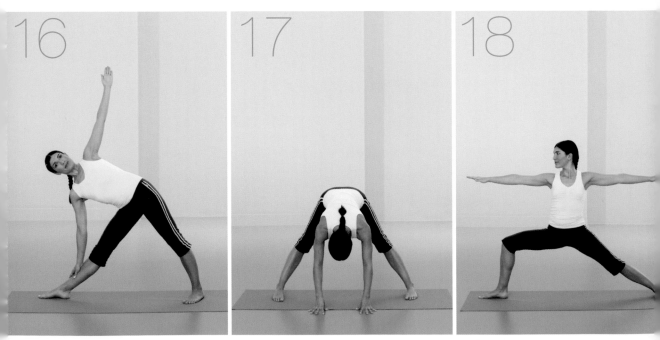

▲ **Triangle**, page 53

▲ **Forward Bend**, page 54

▲ **Warrior 2**, page 54

strengthening at a glance

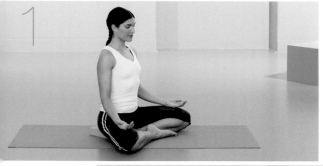

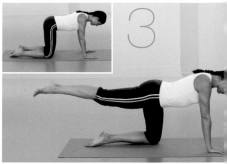

▲ **Quieting the mind**, page 46

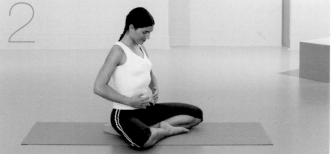

▲ **Shining Skull** (Kapalabhati), page 46

▲ **Diagonal Stretch**, page 47

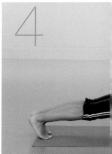

▲ **Plank**, page 47

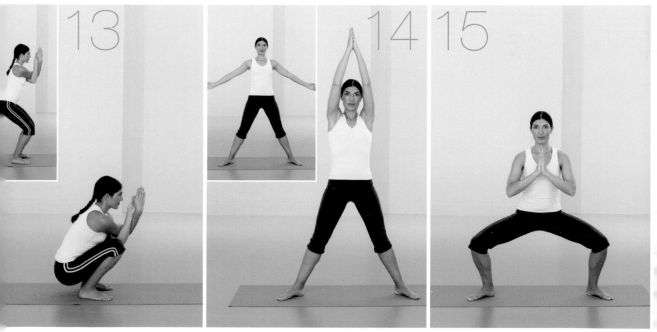

▲ **Squat**, page 52

▲ **Preparation for Horse**, page 52

▲ **Horse**, page 53

strengthening >>

>> **strengthening** FAQs

The Strengthening sequence is designed to improve balance and strengthen your entire body. As a beginner, you may find that some of the poses are difficult at first. Build your strength gradually and take notice of the following advice. Over time, you may feel stronger, taller, and more grounded, and it may become easier to perform everyday activities.

>> What is Kapalabhati?

This breathing exercise is one of the *kriyas* (purifying exercises). It clears the lungs of stale air, making way for a fresh intake of oxygen-rich air and cleans the entire respiratory system. It is wonderfully invigorating and uplifting, clearing the mind and helping to enhance concentration, hence the translation, Shining Skull. The movement of the diaphragm also aids healthier digestion. You can increase the number of rounds when you feel more practiced. It is quite common to feel light-headed during or after this exercise; just return to normal breathing.

>> I can't balance in the Diagonal Stretch. What should I do?

It can be difficult to balance when you first begin and it is very important that you do not feel pain in your lower back. Start by stretching just one arm forward and then the other arm, then stretch one leg back and then the other leg until you become stronger in the central axis and feel able to stretch alternate legs and arms together.

>> I find the Plank very difficult. Any advice?

The Plank develops core strength and stability and strengthens the muscles of the arms, shoulders, and spine. Initially, if you find it hard, just lift for half a second and then release. When you are lifting off the floor, push away with your heels and feel the muscles in your legs wrapping around the bones. Keep your shoulders away from your ears and feel an imaginary string behind your navel, pulling it back to your spine. Once you start to shake, rest, and then do another. Build up gradually over time and stop if you experience any lower back pain.

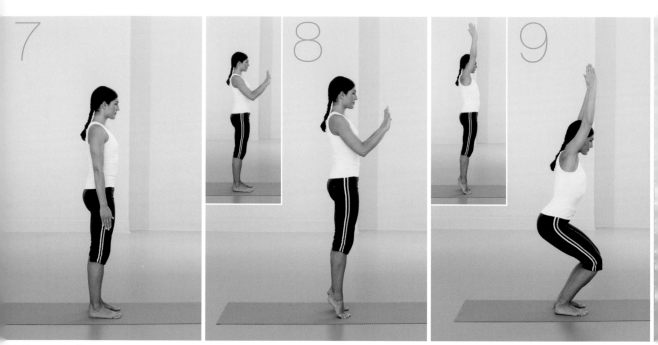

▲ **Mountain Pose**, page 49

▲ **Tiptoes**, page 49

▲ **Chair Pose**, page 50

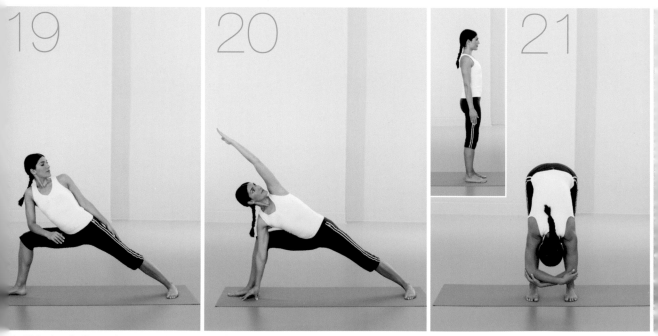

▲ **Side Angle Stretch**, page 55

▲ **Side Angle Stretch**, page 55

▲ **Standing Forward Bend**, page 56

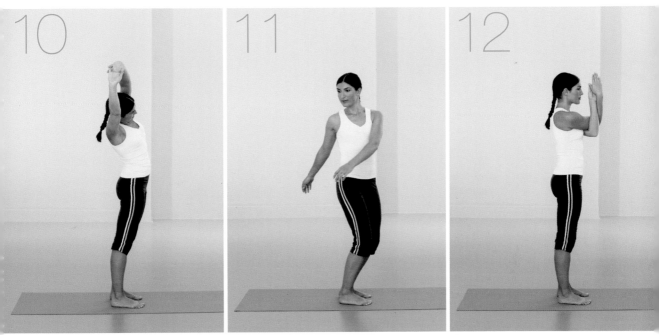

▲ **Standing Lateral Stretch**, page 50   ▲ **Standing Rhythmic Twist**, page 51   ▲ **Eagle Arms**, page 51

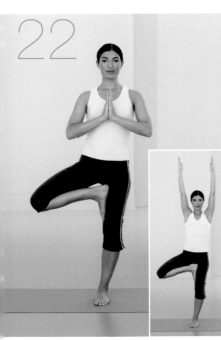

▲ **Tree Pose**, page 56

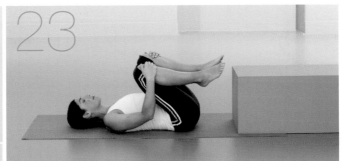

▲ **Final Relaxation**, Back Release, page 57

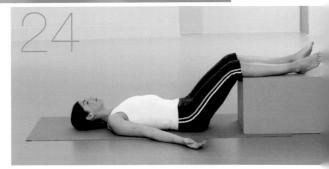

▲ **Final Relaxation**, page 57

15 minute **summary**

I feel heavy and uncomfortable in the Downward Dog, even when I bend my knees. Please help.

Downward Dog livens up the body, but it is more complex than it looks. It demands a balanced effort from the arms, legs, and torso and stretches and strengthens the whole body. If you find the Dog difficult at first, start with the Half Dog. Place your hands on the seat of a chair (against a wall, to prevent it from slipping). This will enable you to straighten your legs more easily. Shoot your buttocks up to the ceiling as you lengthen down the back of your legs to your heels. Feel the front of your thigh lifting up into your groin. Once you feel practiced in the Half Dog, return to the full Downward Dog, but bend your knees to help take the weight back into the legs (see Step 5, p48). Shoot your buttocks up and work your heels down, feeling the extension in your spine. To help lengthen the hamstrings, bend one leg as you stretch the other and alternate. Then try the full pose (p25).

What do you mean by "change the interlace of your fingers" in the Standing Lateral Stretch?

For Step 10, your fingers are interlaced with the pads of your fingers resting on the top of your other hand and your thumbs crossed. When you change the interlace, move the fingers of one hand along one, toward your thumb, so that your other index finger is now in front and your other thumb is crossed on top. If you are a newcomer to yoga, you may notice a great difference between the two and the second version may feel a little odd, but after you have been practicing for a while, they both feel balanced.

How do I prevent myself from falling over in the Tree Pose?

The Tree Pose is a balance pose that opens up the hips and strengthens the legs. It is often taught very early on to beginners because it shows people just how uneven they are and how hard it is to balance. If you find it difficult to balance, put your back against a wall and use it for support or stand near a shelf for you to hold onto if you lose your balance (see p15). Focusing on a stationary point in front of you will help you maintain your balance. If your foot keeps on slipping down from your inner thigh, wrap a belt around your ankle and hold the belt with your hand. If you cannot bring your foot onto your inner thigh, simply place it lower down your leg.

15 minute

Clear your mind
and ease away the
tensions of a hectic
and stressful day

early evening
energizer >>

>> **early evening** energizer

After a long day at work, this routine helps us find the energy to get through the evening. By opening the shoulders and chest and mobilizing the spine, it eases the stress of sitting for hours hunched over a desk, and also helps clear the mind of the day's clutter.

As with all the sequences in this book, don't progress to the stronger stretches until your body is ready. If you feel any compression or pinching in your lower back, remain on the easier versions. Some of the postures in this sequence may seem impossible at first, so be patient and take longer practicing fewer postures more slowly until you feel no back pain, only a good, lengthening stretch.

The exercises

We begin with a period of silent sitting, which allows your mind to clear the thoughts of the day. Feel the firmness of the floor beneath your sitbones anchor your body, allowing the spine to lengthen, and the upper body to rest free from tension. Bringing your thumb and index fingers to meet provides another focus for a scattered mind as you tune into your breath. If the the energy-balancing Alternate Nostril Breathing is a strain, practice the hand position throughout the day and, at first, just do one round before resting, gradually building up your practice.

If your knees feel stiff in the kneeling poses, place a folded blanket at the back of your knees and a block under your buttocks. If your ankles hurt, a folded blanket or two beneath your shins or a rolled towel under the ankles will also help.

The arm exercises ease stiffness and increase flexibility in the shoulders. Imagine the energy extending all along the outside of your body, and ease off if you experience sharp pains in your upper arms. The postures then encourage flexibility in stiff

> ## >> **tips for** early evening energizer
>
> - **Sitting on the floor** for the breathing sequences may be difficult if you are new to yoga. Instead, practice standing or sitting on a firm chair with your back straight.
>
> - **In all the mini-backbends** you should feel no pain in your lower back. If you do, see p89 for advice.
>
> - **In the Quadriceps Stretch**, aim to achieve a strong stretch along the front of the thigh, but release the intensity if you feel any pain in your knee or lower back. Try to keep your hip bones parallel as you stretch.

hips and thighs. In the Lunge, place a support under your back knee, if necessary, to allow you gradually to increase the stretch, energizing the legs and pelvis.

Increasing flexibility and strengthening the back is the final focus of the sequence. Enjoy the safety of the Diagonal Stretch until you feel up to the stronger back bends, and soothe the lower back by ending in Child's Pose and the twisting counterposes.

The energizing Lord of the Fishes Twist is a wonderful antidote to a hunched, deskbound day, relieving any neck and upper back tension and improving posture.

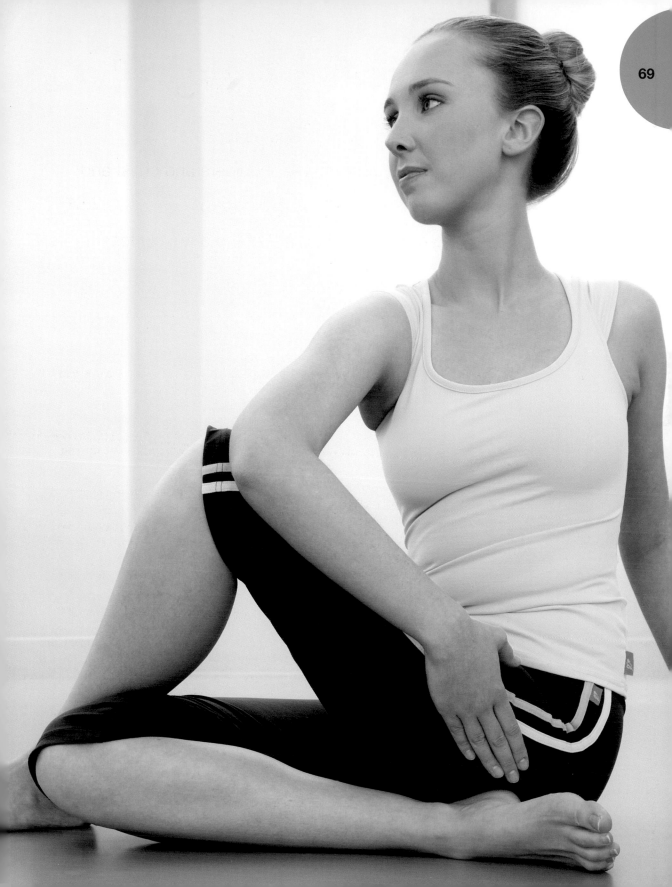

>> **energizer** alternate nostril breathing

1 Sit cross-legged, ready for **Alternate Nostril Breathing**. Rest your hands on your thighs with your palms facing upward. Bring the tips of your index fingers and thumbs together for **Chin Mudra**. Close your eyes and watch your natural breath.

eyes closed

index finger and thumb touching

2 On your right hand, bend the index and middle fingers down (see top inset), so that your thumb is free to close your right nostril, and your ring and little fingers are together, ready to close your left nostril. Inhale through both nostrils. Block your right nostril (see bottom inset). Exhale through the left for 4 counts. Inhale through the left for 4 counts. Change, blocking the left nostril. Exhale through the right. Inhale through the right. Change and exhale through the left to complete a full round. Do 2 more rounds.

>> **energizer** kneeling poses

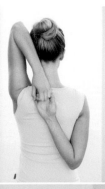

easier option

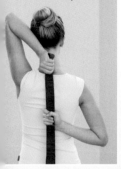

3 Come up to kneeling and bring your arms into **Cow Face** pose. Take your right hand behind and up your back. Bring your left arm up by your head, bending the elbow so that your forearm comes down your back to clasp the fingers of your right hand. If this is difficult, use a belt (see easier option). Feel your abdomen drawing back to the spine to support your lower back. Stay for a couple of breaths. Release your arms and repeat on the other side.

4 Stay kneeling, but tuck your toes under and sit on your heels. Exhale and interlace your fingers, stretching your arms out in front of you. Inhale and lift your arms up over your head, keeping them straight. It is common for the toes to hurt a little here, but you should not experience any knee pain. Stay in this pose for just a few seconds at first.

hands reaching up

head is straight

elbows are stretching away from each other

abdomen is drawing back to the spine

sitbones down on your heels

>> **energizer** kneeling pose/shoulder rolls

5 Exhale, releasing your hands. With your left hand on your right thigh and your right hand behind you on your left buttock, twist to the right. Inhale, moving back to the center. Change the interlace of your fingers and repeat Steps 4 and 5, twisting to the left. If your toes are too painful, put your feet flat again and build up gradually to sitting on your heels.

6 Still kneeling, put your feet flat again. Inhale and move your shoulders forward and up. Exhale, moving them back and down. Repeat twice more. Reverse, moving back and up as you inhale and forward and down as you exhale. Repeat twice more.

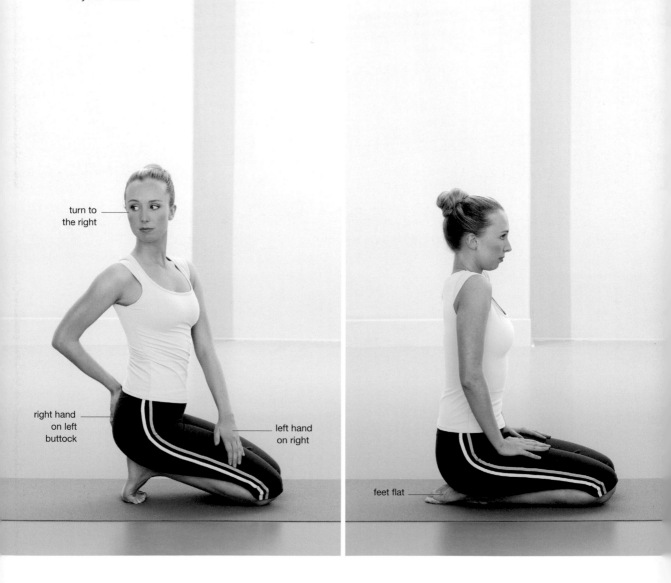

turn to the right

right hand on left buttock

left hand on right

feet flat

7 Come up onto all-fours with your hands in line with your shoulders and your knees in line with your hips. Keep your neck long and your shoulders broad and away from your ears. Feel your abdomen drawing back to the spine.

abdomen drawing back to the spine

knees in line with hips

hands in line with shoulders

8 Step your right foot forward in between your hands for **Lunge**. Keep your front shin perpendicular to the floor. If your back knee is hurting on the floor, place a folded towel under it. Sink your hips, stretching your back leg more.

stretch your leg back

fingers touching floor

>> **energizer** lunge/downward dog

9 Bring both hands onto your front knee. Exhale, increasing the stretch on your back leg. Feel a strong stretch on your back thigh. Inhale, placing your hands on the floor by your front foot. Exhale and come back onto all-fours. Repeat on the other side. Come back onto all-fours.

shoulders down and broad

feel a strong stretch on your quadricep

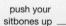

10 Inhale, tucking your toes under. Exhale, drawing your abdomen toward your spine and lifting your pelvis to form an inverted "V" with your body in the **Downward Dog**. Keep your arms and legs straight and turn your armpits to face each other. Push your buttocks up and stretch back and down with your heels, keeping your breath even and smooth.

push your sitbones up

keep legs straight, if possible

keep arms straight

>> **energizer** diagonal stretch

11 Inhale and come back onto your knees. Exhale and lie on your stomach with your forehead on the floor and your arms stretched out in front of you.

12 Exhale, lifting and stretching your right arm and left leg and bringing your head just off the floor. Inhale, bring them back down to the floor. Exhale and repeat on your other side. Repeat again on both sides. Make sure you stretch all along the inside of your leg to the heel. As you stretch your arm forward, keep your shoulders away from your ears.

shoulders away from your ears and broad

>> **energizer** rest/locust

13 Rest. Place your arms by your side with your palms by your hips, facing upward. Turn your head to one side. Lie with your big toes touching and your heels facing out. Close your eyes and focus on even, gentle breathing.

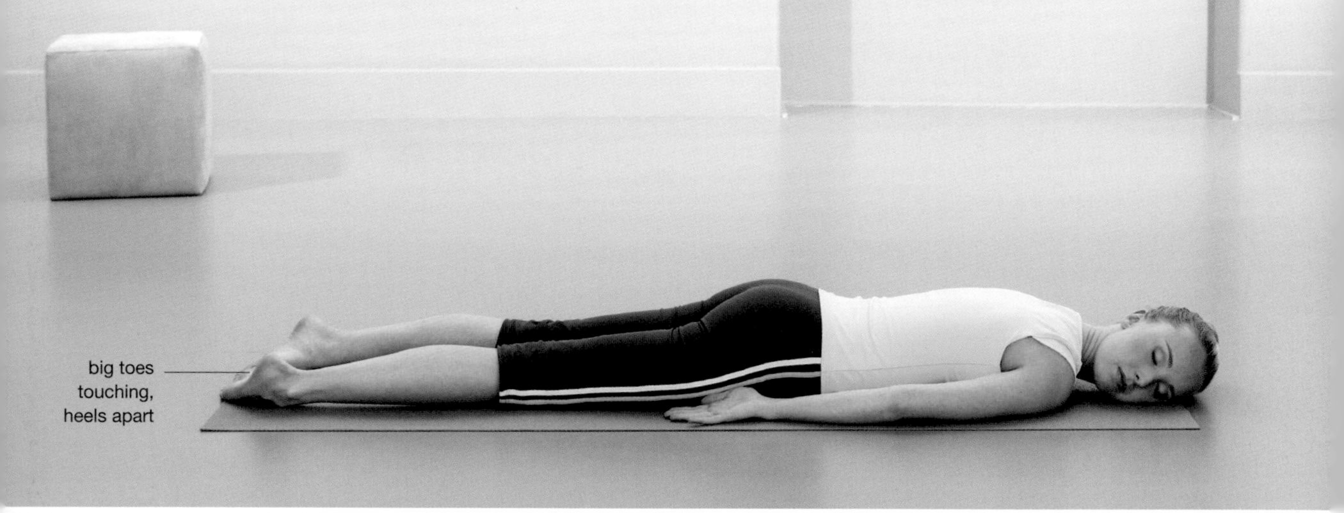

big toes
touching,
heels apart

14 Inhale, bringing your head back to the center. Stretch your hands back toward your toes. Keep your feet and legs firmly on the floor as you exhale, peeling your nose, chin, head and shoulders off the floor in the **Locust** pose. Breathe evenly. As long as there is no pain in your lower back, lift a little higher. Inhale and relax your body down.

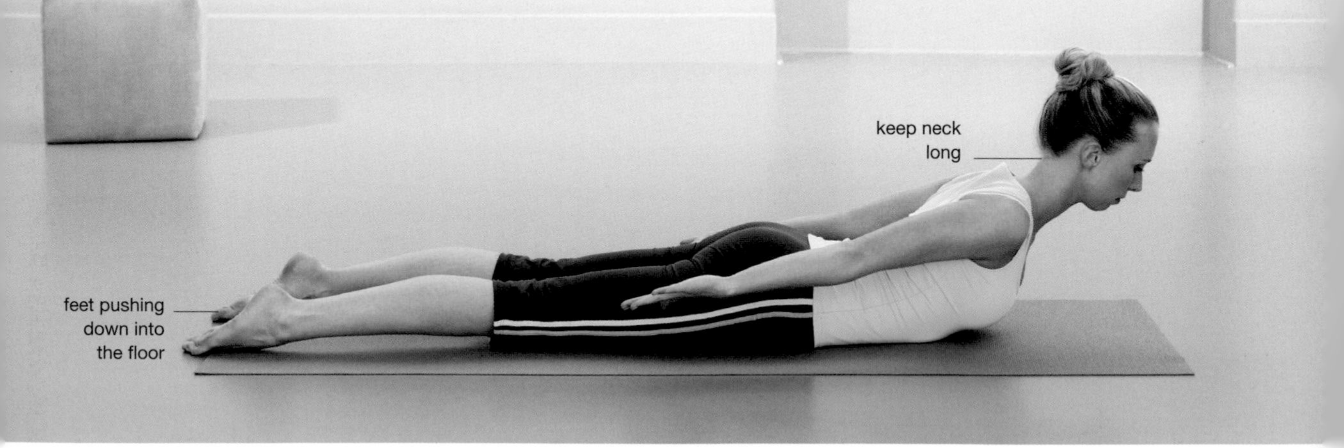

keep neck
long

feet pushing
down into
the floor

15 If you want to work a little harder, exhale, lifting your straight legs as well as your head and shoulders off the floor. Stretch your arms back toward your feet. Inhale and come down. Repeat (as long as you are not experiencing any back pain).

stretch your arms back toward your feet

16 Rest, as you did in Step 13, but turn your head the other way. For a **Quadriceps Stretch**, place your left forearm on the floor in front of you. Lift your head. Bend your right leg and, with your right hand on top of your right foot, stretch your right foot down toward the floor on the outside of your right hip. Breathe evenly.

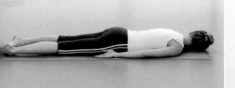

forearm rests horizontally in front of you

pubic bone pushing into the floor

navel lifting toward your chest

>> **energizer** half bow/rest

17 Inhale and move your hand to hold the outside of your right ankle, ready for a **Half Bow**. Keep both hip bones on the floor. Exhale and lift your right thigh up off the floor. Breathe evenly. Inhale and release down. Repeat Steps 16 and 17 on your left side.

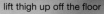

lift thigh up off the floor | keep hip bones on the floor

18 Make a pillow with your hands in front of you and rest your forehead on your hands. Lie with your big toes touching and your heels apart. Rest, breathing gently.

big toes touching

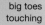

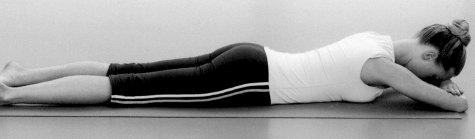

easier option

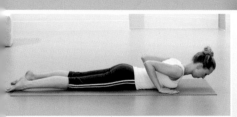

19 To do the **Full Bow**, bend both knees up and hold your ankles firmly with your hands. Exhale and lift your thighs up off the floor. Inhale and, as long as there is no pain in your lower back, lift a little higher as you exhale. Inhale and come down. Use a belt if you find this difficult (see inset).

20 Bring your hands under your shoulders, exhale, and push back into **Child's Pose**. Your heels are apart and your big toes are touching. Bring your head to the floor and feel your buttocks stretching down toward your heels. Bring your hands by your feet with your palms facing upward. Breathe in and feel the breath move in your lower back. Exhale and release your buttocks back and down toward your heels. Follow your natural breath.

palms facing upward

forehead on the floor

>> **energizer** lord of the fishes twist

21 Inhale, rolling up vertebra by vertebra, with your head coming up last, until you are sitting on your heels. To do the **Lord of the Fishes Twist**, sit on your left side with your feet out to the right. Place your right foot on the floor, on the outside of your left knee. Rest your left elbow on your right knee. Inhale and feel yourself getting taller. Exhale and turn to the right. Inhale and feel yourself getting taller. Exhale and turn to the right.

right hand on floor behind you

sitbones push down

easier option

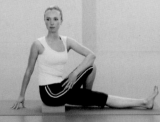

22 Inhale and come back to the center. Repeat on your other side. If you find this twist difficult, place a block underneath you and stretch one leg out in front of you, crossing your other leg over it, bringing the opposite elbow round the top knee (see easier option). Inhale and come back to the center. Release your legs out in front of you.

twist as far as possible

fingers touching the floor or block

foot flat on floor

23 Lie flat on your back and check that you are straight. Place your right foot behind your left knee. Hold your right thigh with your left hand as you take your right knee toward the floor on the left. Looking out toward the right, let your right arm release to the floor and feel the stretch through your right shoulder and armpit. Inhale and come back to center. Release your legs and repeat on your other side (see inset).

turn head to
the right

right foot is behind
left knee

24 Inhale and come back to the center. Lie flat with your knees bent and your feet on the floor (hip-width apart and parallel). Lift your head and look down your center line to see that you are straight. Place your head on the floor and your arms away from your body. Lengthen one leg out along the floor and then the other, ready for the Final Relaxation. Close your eyes and stay here for 2–5 minutes. Place a folded blanket under your head, a cushion under your knees and an eye pad on your eyes, if you wish, to make you more comfortable.

shoulders relaxed
and away from ears

palms facing upward

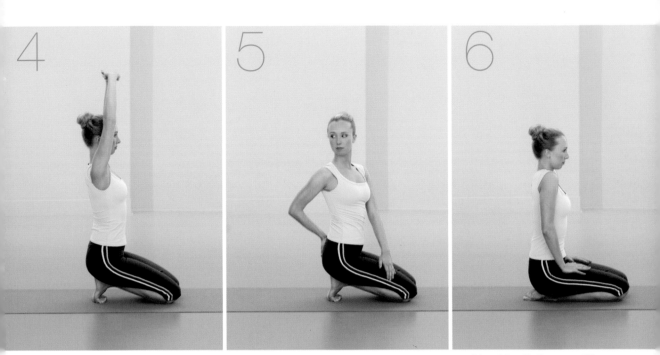

▲ **Kneeling Pose**, interlacing, page 71

▲ **Kneeling Pose**, Twist, page 72

▲ **Shoulder Rolls**, page 72

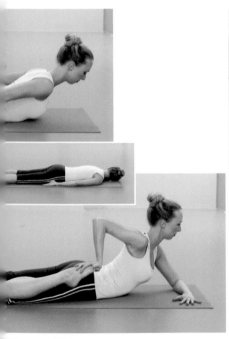

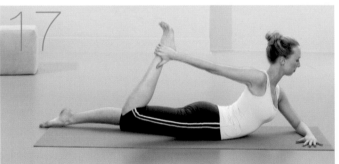

▲ **Half Bow**,
page 78

ch, page 77

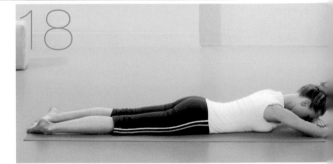

▲ **Rest**, page 78

energizer at a glance

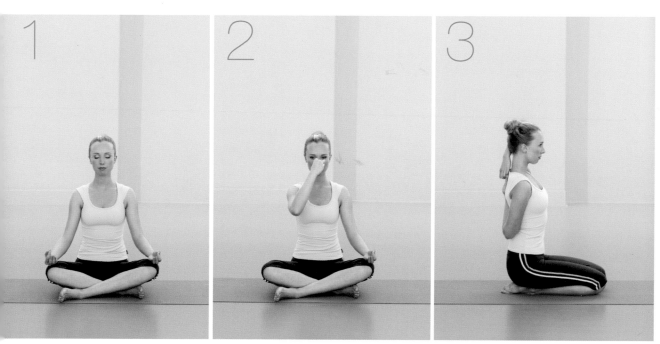

▲ **Chin Mudra**, page 70   ▲ **Alternate Nostril Breathing**, page 70   ▲ **Kneeling Pose**, Cow Face, page 71

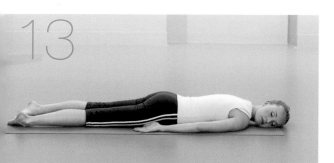

▲ **Rest**,
page 76

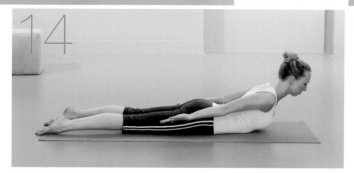

▲ **Locust**, page 76

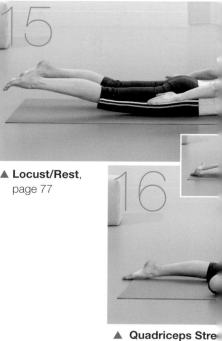

▲ **Locust/Rest**,
page 77

▲ **Quadriceps Stre**

early evening energizer >>

>> energizer FAQs

Some of the poses in this sequence look deceptively simple, so do not feel discouraged if you are unable to carry out the full pose at first. You are still benefiting from the stretch. Remember, yoga is not a competition. Read the following tips to improve your practice and to make you more comfortable.

>> What is Chin Mudra?

A *mudra* is a gesture or seal that we make with our hands or another part of the body. The most well-known *mudra* is *Chin Mudra*. The tip of the thumb and the index finger lightly touch each other, representing the individual and Higher Self uniting. The other three fingers gently stretch out and the back of the hand or palm rests on the thigh or knee. It gives you another focus point to help you stay in the present moment while you are performing a breathing exercise or meditating.

>> What do I do if I cannot breathe through my nose in the Alternate Nostril Breathing exercise?

Alternate nostril breathing is believed to calm the mind and nervous system. It should not, however, be practiced if you have a cold or your nose is very blocked. If your nose is a little blocked, take one breath at a time through your nose, then breathe through your mouth again, and repeat. You can manipulate your nostrils by bringing your fingers up to the bridge of your nose to open the nostrils further. Take it easy, do not cause pressure, and do not force it.

>> I find Cow Face pose particularly hard. Any tips?

Our shoulders are often very stiff, but this pose can help release any stiff muscles there. Often one shoulder is stiffer than the other. Make a swimming breaststroke movement, bringing your lower arm up your back, gently manipulating your hand farther up your back. Stand near a wall and let the lower arm's elbow push into the wall to encourage your hand farther up your back. If your hands are very far from reaching each other, use a belt to help you (see easier option, Step 3, p71). With practice, you will be able to clasp your fingers together.

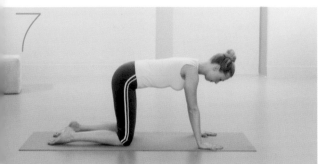

▲ **All-Fours**, page 73

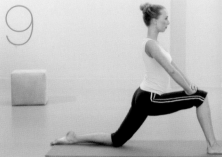

▲ **Lunge**, page 74

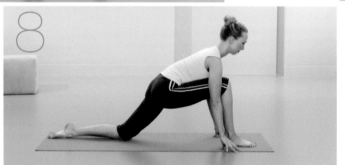

▲ **Lunge**, page 73

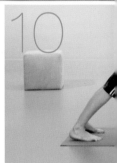

▲ **Downward Dog**,

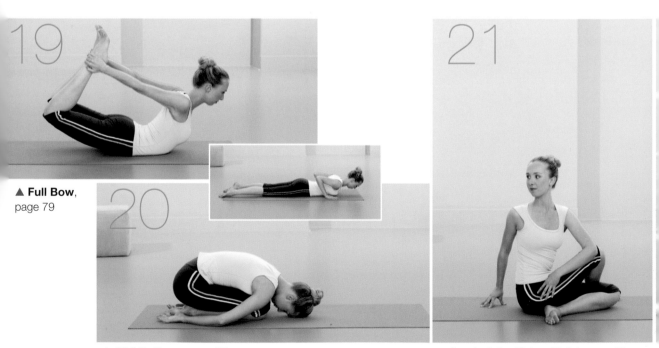

▲ **Full Bow**, page 79

▲ **Child's Pose**, page 79

▲ **Lord of the Fishes Twist**, page 80

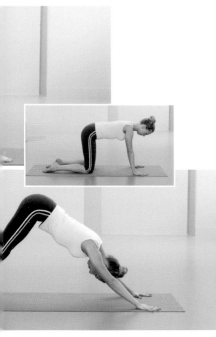

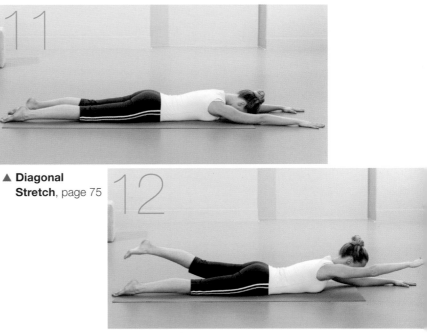

▲ **Diagonal Stretch**, page 75

page 74

▲ **Diagonal Stretch**, page 75

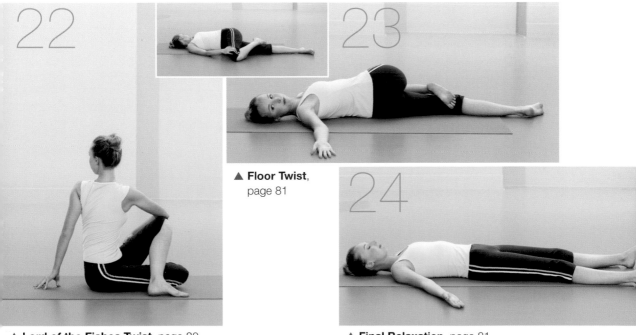

▲ **Floor Twist**, page 81

▲ **Lord of the Fishes Twist**, page 80

▲ **Final Relaxation**, page 81

15 minute **summary**

>> I found that my lower back hurt during the Locust. What should I do to stop this?

Stop immediately if you are experiencing any lower back pain. If your lower back is sensitive, do not go further than Step 14 (p76), the single arm and leg Locust. Feel like you are in traction with your hands being pulled forward and your feet backward. Feel a lengthening and strength in your arms and legs. Push your pubic bone down into the floor. Breathe evenly. Only practice the Locust if you are no longer experiencing any pain, otherwise stay with Step 14.

>> The Quadriceps Stretch hurts. Is this normal?

Tight quadriceps make bending your back harder and it puts more strain on the hamstrings. It is therefore important to regularly stretch them gently. Often they really sting, but continue; this is positive pain. At first, if your quadriceps are so tight that you cannot hold your foot with your hand, place a belt around your ankle and bring your foot down toward the outside of your hip. If you do this regularly, you will notice a real difference and you may also find that your posture improves as you stand up straighter. At first, if you find it difficult to lift your head, simply rest it on your front hand or arm.

>> I find Child's Pose uncomfortable. Can you give me some advice?

Although at first this may not seem like a very comfortable position to be in, it becomes a favorite of many, since it calms breathing and helps settle the mind and body, providing a gentle way to deeply relax. The key is to find ways to just let your weight go and still be comfortable. If you find it uncomfortable to let your weight rest on your lower legs, place a folded blanket between your thighs and calves. This will tilt you forward and can allow you to relax and let your weight drop. If you find your buttocks are not touching your heels, you can also place a folded blanket under your buttocks to make yourself more comfortable. On every exhalation, release your buttocks back down toward your heels and over time, your buttocks will rest on your heels. If your head is not touching the floor, you can make fists with your hands and place one fist on top of the other and rest your forehead on the top fist.

15 minute

winding
down >>

Watch your breath become slower and deeper as you prepare for a restful night's sleep

>> **winding** down

This sequence is designed to quiet your body and mind and ready you for deep, restorative sleep. If you find you are still wakeful, shift any remaining tension by lying on your back, repeating the Bound Angle or Bridge poses and watching your breathing become slower and deeper.

If you do not have time for the whole sequence, just lie in the final relaxation, or Corpse pose and systematically tense and release every part of your body in turn. Start with your feet and work up through your legs, buttocks, hands and arms, chest and shoulders, and finally your face. This teaches your body how to let go of its armor of physical tension and helps you release unhelpful or negative thought patterns.

The exercises

This sequence begins with mind-calming forward bends. Just relax and let gravity and the out-breath do the work for you—imagine it divesting you of thoughts and concerns. If your knees will not straighten, raise your buttocks on blocks or folded blankets, or sit with your back against a wall and listen to your breath. To stop your back from hunching, loop a belt around the foot of your straight leg, taking one end in each hand. On the inhale, pull on the belt to help you sit tall; on the exhale, hinge forward, aiming to walk your hands down the belt toward your foot. Do not struggle to get your head down—it doesn't matter if you never manage to bend forward. Instead, focus on sitting tall to strengthen the lower back and lengthen the hamstrings, cushioning the thigh of your bent leg if your knee doesn't reach the floor. If even this feels onerous, just lie on your back with your legs crossed.

To relax your lower back after forward bending, lie on your back, drawing your knees into your chest. Then practice pelvic-floor lifts: lift the

> ## >> **tips for** winding down
>
> - **Forward bends** may be easiest at first if you place a chair in front of you and simply relax your forehead onto its seat.
>
> - **Hinging from the hips** is essential in forward bending. If this seems tricky, tilt your pelvis forward by placing blocks beneath your buttocks to stop your back from hunching.
>
> - **For the Bridge,** make sure the height beneath your buttocks feels comfortable so that your back remains unstrained. Rest your head and shoulders on the floor.

muscles between your genitals and anus as you exhale and release as you inhale. Progress to the supported Bridge pose: lying with your chest open and outer shoulders and upper arms on the floor is quieting and calming. Lower your back down slowly, taking one block out at a time, and let the twists ease out any tightness before lying in Corpse pose and just letting go. If you wish, raise your calves on a chair or put a bolster under your knees.

Enjoy the Side Angle Stretch, relishing the long extension from your hip to fingertips as it eases out any residual tension of the day.

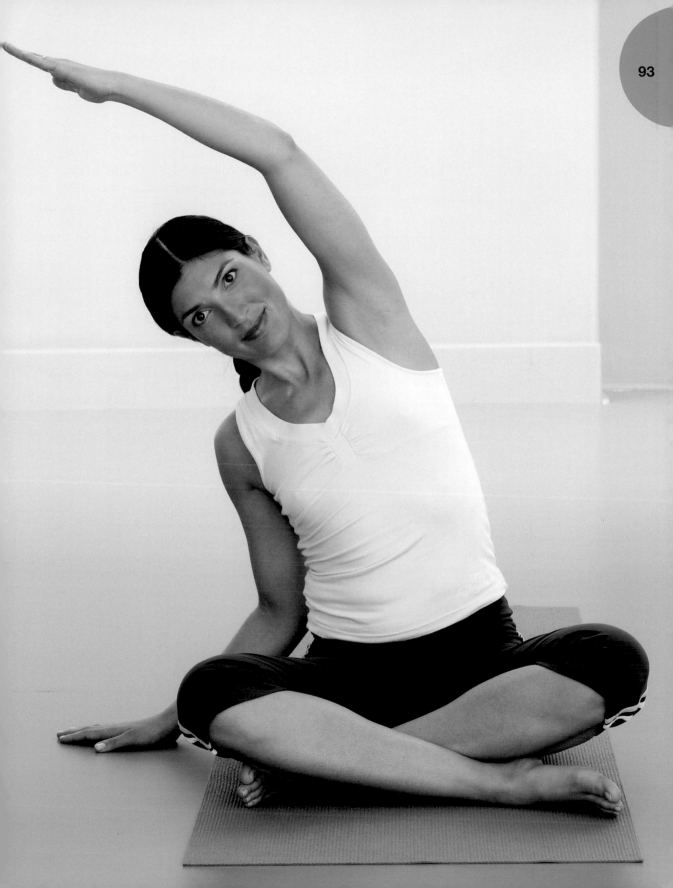

>> **winding down** bound angle/neck rolls

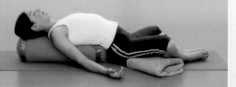

easier option

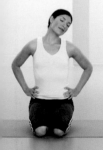

1 Lie flat on your back with the soles of your feet together for **Bound Angle Pose**. If you like, place blankets and a bolster underneath you to help open your chest (see inset). Close your eyes and follow a breathing circuit: breathe in and wash the brain with the inhalation. Exhale down your spine to your tailbone. Inhale up your spine to in between your eyebrows. Exhale through both your nostrils. Repeat this circuit once more.

soles of feet together

arms away from body, palms facing upward

2 Roll to the side and come up to sitting on your heels. Place your hands on your waist for **Neck Rolls**. Imagine you are drawing a circle with the crown of the head. Bring your chin down toward your chest. Inhale as you move your head to the right and back. Exhale as you move to the left and forward. Repeat and then reverse.

if your neck feels tight, make the circles smaller

hands on waist

easier option

3 Release your legs forward and sit cross-legged. Push down and back with your sitbones and extend your torso over your thighs. Put your hands on the floor in front of you. With each exhalation, stretch forward with your fingers and push down and back with your sitting bones. Breathe naturally. If it is too difficult to come forward, lie on your back with your legs crossed (see inset).

shoulders relaxed and
away from your ears

inch forward on
each exhalation

4 Inhale and come back up for a **Side Angle Stretch**. Place your right hand on the floor by your right hip. Keep your elbow bent and shoulder relaxed. Inhale and sweep your left arm up and over your head. Exhale, feeling the stretch on your left side. Inhale and exhale, feeling the stretch. Keep your breathing relaxed. Inhale and come back to the center. Repeat on the other side.

keep head
relaxed

sitbones firm on
the floor

5 Inhale and change the cross of your legs. Relax forward again, as your sitbones push down and back and your fingers inch forward on every exhalation. Let go. On each exhalation, let your torso hinge forward over your thighs to open the hips. If your knees hurt, push back and down with your buttocks and do not come so far forward.

inch forward
on every
exhalation

root down and back

6 Inhale and come up. Place your left hand on your right thigh and your right hand on the floor behind you, and turn your head and torso to the right. As you inhale, feel yourself getting taller. Exhale, twisting. Inhale and come back to the center. Repeat on the left side.

turn head and torso
to the right

7 Release your legs out in front of you. Bend your right knee and place your foot against the inside of your left thigh. If your knee is not resting on the floor, place a support under the thigh. Keep your left leg straight. Inhale, sit up, and look forward. Place your fingers on the floor behind you. Exhale and come down over your straight leg, bringing your hands to the floor on either side of your leg (see inset). Inhale and come up. Release your right leg out and repeat on the other side.

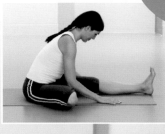

feel even weight
through your hands

8 Inhale and come up. Stretch both legs out in front of you. Place your hands on the floor behind you. Sit up. As you push down with your sitbones, feel yourself getting taller. Sit on a support if your back is weak and hold a belt around your feet to help you sit up straight.

>> **winding down** seated forward bend

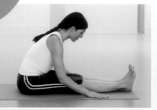

9 Move your hands forward on either side of your legs, as you hinge forward at your hips (see inset). Feel an even weight through both hands. On every exhalation, coming down until, over time, you can clasp both feet.

legs straight

10 Inhale, come up, and lie flat on the floor. With your hands clasped around your knees, hug your knees toward your body. Lift your pelvic floor muscles. As you exhale, lift the pelvic floor. As you inhale, release. Repeat several times.

knees hugged toward body

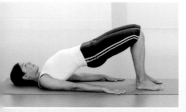

11 Place your feet flat on the floor, hip-width apart. Place your arms on the floor, stretching toward your feet.
As you exhale, peel your lower back off the floor, lifting your hips and chest up as your feet grow roots down (see inset). This is the **Bridge** pose. Place the blocks under your hips.
If your back hurts, place fewer blocks beneath you and lengthen your tailbone toward your knees.

feet, knees, and legs parallel

feet flat

head and shoulders on the floor

12 Stay as you are, with your hips heavy on the blocks, your chest lifting, and your feet firm on the floor. If there is any pain in your lower back, take a block out. If you want to go further, bend your right knee toward your chest and stretch your right leg straight up. Your left foot remains firm on the floor and your hips are even. Breathe naturally. Inhale and bring your right foot back down to the floor. Repeat with your left leg.

straight leg, reaching up to the ceiling

foot flat on the floor and straight

>> **winding down** bridge/floor twist

13 If you want to go further, bend both knees toward your chest and stretch both legs straight up. Your hips are heavy on the blocks and your chest is lifting. Return your feet to the floor. Lift your hips off the blocks and take the blocks out, slowly releasing your back down to the floor. Hug your knees toward your chest.

chest lifting

hips heavy on blocks

14 Stretch your legs out in front of you for a **Floor Twist**. Wrap your right leg over your left leg and take both legs down to the floor on your left, holding your right thigh with your left hand. Release your right arm out to the side. Look toward your right shoulder and, with every exhalation, stretch your right arm out a little more. If your right arm is high off the floor, rest it on a cushion to help you release. Inhale as you come back to the center. Repeat to the right.

bring legs down to the floor

arm out at 45 degrees to your body

>> **winding down** final relaxation

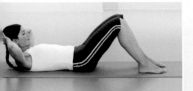

15 Get ready for the **Final Relaxation**. Lie on the floor with your knees bent and feet flat. Place your hands under your head and lift your head to look down your center line (see inset). Gently lay your head back down on the floor. Bring your arms out a little way from your body with your palms facing upward. Stretch one leg out and then the other leg out along the floor.

shoulders relaxed, away from ears

16 Lie straight and relaxed, with a folded blanket under your head and something to cover you, if you like. Close your eyes. Now you are going to tense and relax each part of your body in turn.

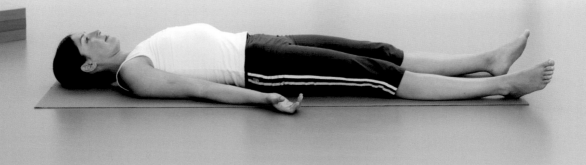

>> **winding down** final relaxation

17 Inhale and lift your right leg slightly off the floor. Tense the leg, exhale, and let it drop to the floor, relaxed. Repeat with your left leg.

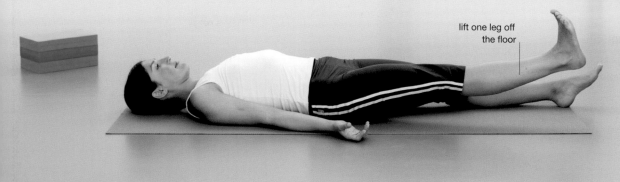

lift one leg off the floor

18 Inhale and lift your hips off the floor as you clench your buttocks together (see inset). Exhale and let them go. Inhale and lift your chest and back off the floor, bringing your shoulder blades together, and keeping your hips and head on the floor. Exhale and relax back down to the floor.

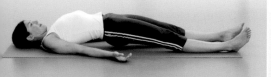

lift chest off the floor

head remains on the floor

hips remain on the floor

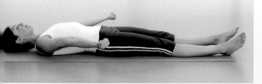

19 Inhale and lift both arms off the floor. Tense your arms, make fists (see inset), then stretch your fingers out. Exhale and let them drop back to the floor.

stretch fingers out

20 Inhale and lift your shoulders, hunching them up tightly toward your ears. Exhale and let them drop, relaxed.

bring shoulders up to ears

>> **winding down** final relaxation

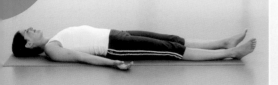

21 Inhale and screw your face up into a tiny ball toward your nose (see inset). Exhale and let go. Open your eyes wide and look backward. Open your mouth, stick your tongue out, and roar. Inhale and release.

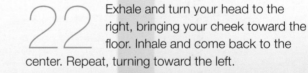

22 Exhale and turn your head to the right, bringing your cheek toward the floor. Inhale and come back to the center. Repeat, turning toward the left.

23 Feel comfortable and symmetrical. Close your eyes and systematically travel through every part of your body, from your toes to your forehead, relaxing every part as you go. Cover your eyes with an eye pad or folded cloth, if you like.

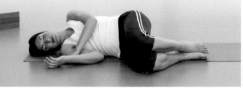

24 When you are ready to come up, roll onto the right side of your body. Stay here for a few seconds and then come up onto all-fours to come up to kneeling. Bring your hands into prayer position, feeling calm and contented, and give thanks.

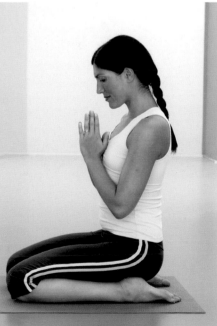

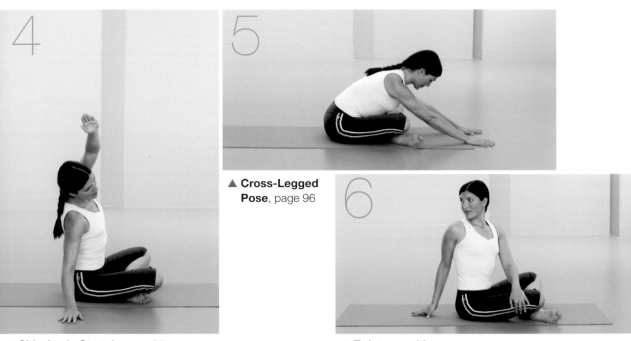

▲ **Side Angle Stretch**, page 95

▲ **Cross-Legged Pose**, page 96

▲ **Twist**, page 96

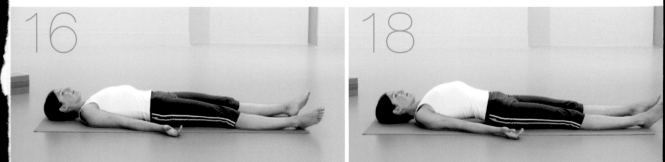

▲ **Final Relaxation**, lie straight, page 101

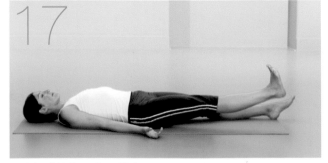

▲ **Final Relaxation**, lift legs, page 102

▲ **Final Relaxation**, lift hips, then chest, page 102

winding down at a glance

1

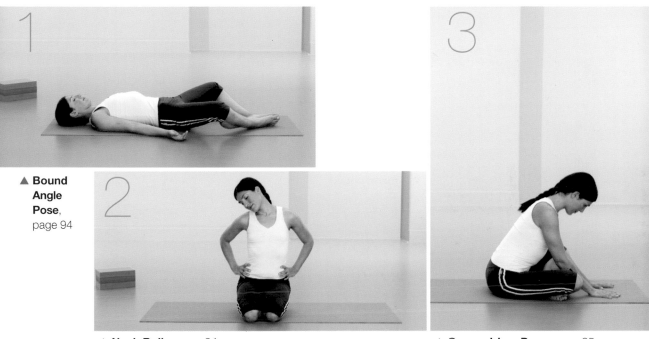

▲ **Bound Angle Pose**, page 94

2

▲ **Neck Rolls**, page 94

3

▲ **Crossed-Leg Pose**, page 95

13

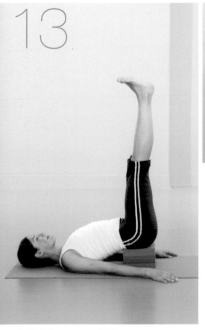

▲ **Bridge**, page 100

14

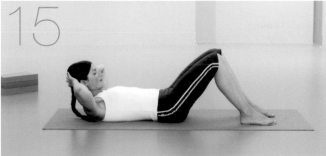

▲ **Floor Twist**, page 100

15

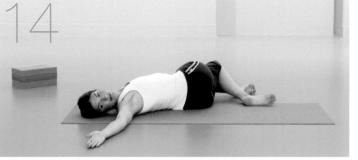

▲ **Final Relaxation**, page 101

winding down >>

15 minute **summary**

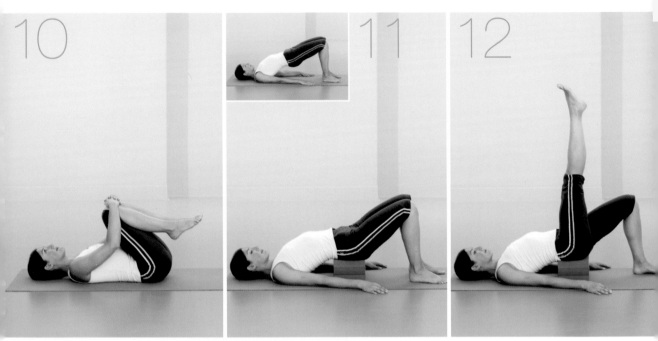

▲ **Hug knees**, page 98

▲ **Bridge**, page 99

▲ **Bridge**, page 99

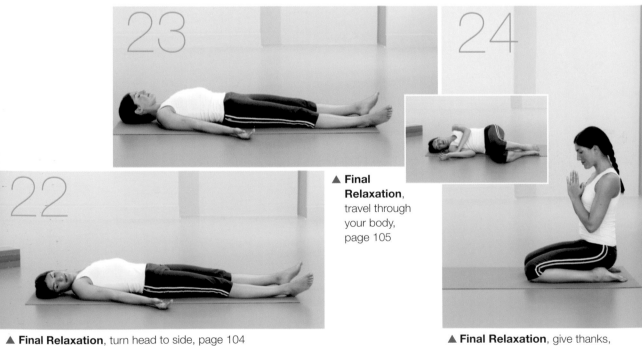

▲ **Final Relaxation**, turn head to side, page 104

▲ **Final Relaxation**, travel through your body, page 105

▲ **Final Relaxation**, give thanks, page 105

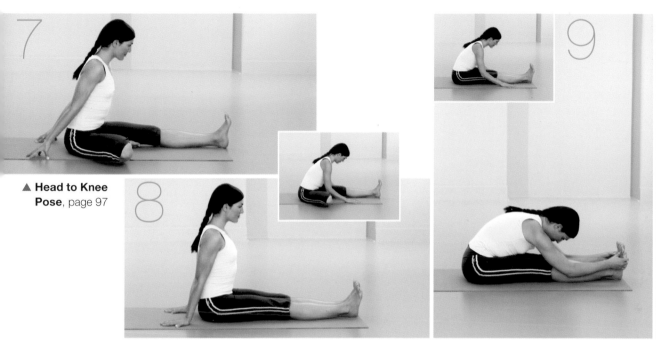

▲ **Head to Knee Pose**, page 97

▲ **Seated Forward Bend**, sitting up straight, page 97

▲ **Seated Forward Bend**, page 98

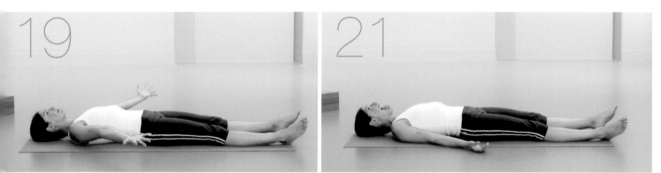

▲ **Final Relaxation,** make fists and stretch fingers out, page 103

▲ **Final Relaxation,** screw face up and stick tongue out, page 104

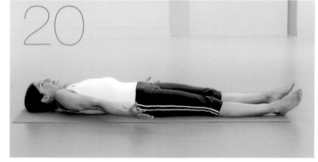

▲ **Final Relaxation**, hunch shoulders, page 103

>> **winding down** FAQs

To actually relax after a stressful day can take time. If you find that you cannot sleep, even after the Final Relaxation, read the following tips below. Some of the poses may be a little hard, particularly if you have tight hamstrings or a stiff neck. If this is the case, take note of the modifications and advice below.

>> **My neck pinches during the Neck Rolls. Is this ok?**

Don't circle your neck if you feel pinches. Instead, bend your neck forward as you exhale and inhale back to the center. Then exhale as you let your head drop backward and inhale, returning to the center. Repeat. Turn your head to the extreme right as you exhale and inhale back to the center. Repeat to the left and repeat once again on both sides. A great advantage of this exercise is that it can be done anywhere—at your desk, while watching television, or while you are washing the dishes. Just a few minutes a day can preserve the neck's elasticity and prevent problems in the future.

>> **What can I do to lengthen my tight hamstrings?**

Tight hamstrings stop you from being able to bend forward in the Head to Knee Pose and the straight-leg Seated Forward Bend. Your hamstrings are the long, powerful muscles at the back of the thigh. Tight hamstrings put the lower back at risk by preventing the pelvis from tilting when you bend forward, making the movement come from the lower back, which is injurious. To lengthen your hamstrings, lie on the floor with your straight legs up against the wall (see p14, bottom right). If your buttocks do not touch the floor or your knees are bent, move farther away from the wall until you can rectify this. This is very relaxing, it drains fluid from the legs, and can help relieve back pain. Doing this for five or 10 minutes every day after work or when you feel particularly exhausted will make a difference. Be gentle with the hamstrings; do not overstretch them. To aid you in the sitting forward bends, place a block under your buttocks and wrap a belt around your feet to help you to sit up.

>> What is my pelvic floor?

These are the band of muscles that, for women, support the urethra, vagina, and rectum, and for men, the penis, bladder, and rectum. To locate them, stop the flow of urine next time you use the toilet; the muscles you use to do this are your pelvic floor. Exercising your pelvic floor is important to build up your core strength. Your pelvic floor muscles should work together efficiently with your abdominal and lower back muscles. Performing pelvic floor exercises regularly helps prevent and overcome incontinence, to prepare for, and recover from, childbirth, and to resolve sexual and erectile dysfunction. This exercise can be performed anywhere, for example, sitting in a traffic jam or at your desk.

>> I don't find the Corpse pose very relaxing. How can I make myself more comfortable?

If you are uncomfortable lying flat on the floor, rest your calves on a chair or stool (as for the Final Relaxation in the Strengthening sequence, p57). You could also place a bolster under your knees and a folded blanket under your head and ankles (see bottom picture, p120). If your eyes flicker, cover them with a folded cloth or eye pad. If you are pregnant, lie on your side.

>> How do I come out of the Final Relaxation?

Come out of the Final Relaxation slowly. Start by wriggling your toes and fingers and then rolling your arms and legs from side to side. Breathe more deeply and stretch your arms over your head, if it feels good to do so. Then roll onto your side and stay there for a little while, using your lower arm as a cushion for your head. Slowly come up onto all-fours, kneel, and then come up to standing.

>> I still feel agitated when I get into bed. What should I do?

After a stressful day, it is sometimes very hard to relax and let go of tension. When lying in bed, go through your body again, tensing and relaxing. You may find covering your eyes with an eye pad or a folded cloth helps. Concentrate on breathing deeply from your abdomen, resting one hand on your abdomen and the other on your chest. After you have been practicing yoga for a while, you should find that you feel less stressed. Try meditation also, to help you let go of your worries and tensions; refer to pp122–123 for advice.

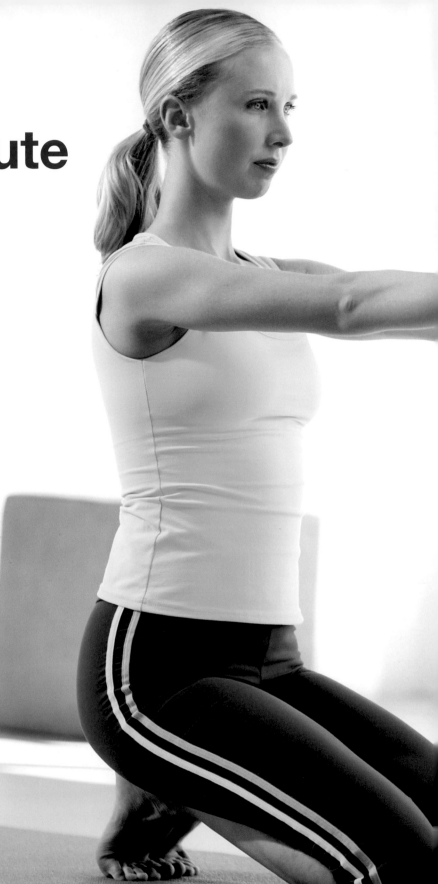

15 minute

all about
yoga >>

Learn more about the history of yoga and how to incorporate yoga into your life

>> **history** of yoga

Yoga developed as a way of living in ancient India's Vedic period, up to four millennia ago. It remains vital today because yogic ways of behaving and thinking answer some fundamental modern questions about health, well-being, and spirituality.

The Sanskrit root of the word "yoga," *yuj*—"to yoke," or "to unite"—helps to explain the system's longevity, for this is a philosophy that shows us how to dissolve conflict and duality, and to bring together body and mind, individual and universal. This union generates an inner peace that not only brings good health and psychological well-being, but reveals spiritual truth. *Hatha* yoga, the physical exercises and breathing practices that this book espouses, also derives its name from a fusion of opposites: it is commonly thought to be a linking of the words for "sun," *ha*, and "moon," *tha*.

Ancient truths

Yoga grew out of an oral tradition: the practices advocated for a yogic way of living were passed down from teacher to student over the centuries until over 2,000 years ago. The Indian sage Patanjali is credited with collating the tradition into the *Yoga Sutras*, a collection of aphorisms generally accepted as the ultimate sourcebook of classical yoga. Patanjali's origins remain shrouded in legend, but he may have been a physician, a scholar of Sanskrit and grammar, and a yogi.

Within the *Yoga Sutras*, Patanjali set out a practical eight-stranded path, which would lead the practitioner toward the ultimate goal of yoga, a true sense of inner peace and communion (see box, opposite). The eight "limbs," or strands, are made up of ethical ways to behave to build a successful society (from not stealing to truthfulness) and personal practices to follow that ensure a righteous

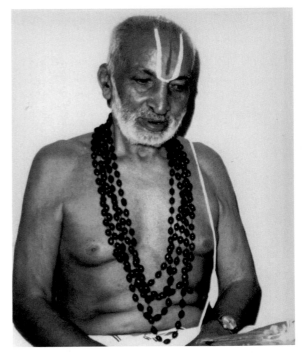

Sri T. Krishnamacharya was 101 when he died and he is often credited as "the father of modern yoga." Some of his leading students went on to popularize yoga in the West.

life (from personal-cleansing regimens to religious devotion). Among these limbs are the practice of yoga's physical postures, *asana*, and its breathing exercises, *pranayama*. The first are advocated as a way of stilling the body to sit in meditation, the latter to ensure a constant supply of *prana*, subtle energy. This remains the path yogis follow today.

Modern gurus

The story of hatha yoga passed into the modern era and out of India largely thanks to the influential teacher Sri Tirumalai Krishnamacharya (1888–1989), who established a school of yoga for boys in the palace of the Maharaja of Mysore, in Karnataka, southern India from the 1920s to the 1950s. In doing so, he brought the ancient but almost forgotten art of yoga to a broader audience in India.

Among Krishnamacharya's pupils were boys who would go on to popularize Patanjali's hatha yoga in the West. From his base in Pune, India, B.K.S. Iyengar (born 1918) developed a form of yoga with appeal for the Western interest in the

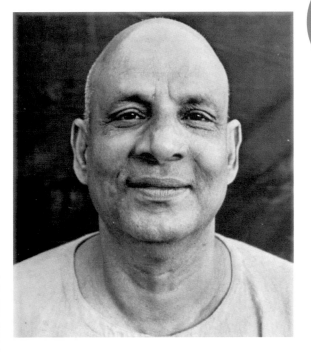

Swami Sivananda was a doctor before renouncing medicine for a spiritual path. At his Ashram in Rishikesh he trained many exceptional disciples in yoga and philosophy.

body, and set up a method of teacher training that ensured his approach would be the most widely practiced across the globe. In Mysore, Sri Pattabhi Jois (born 1915) pursued his teacher's early form of athletic yoga sequences to form *ashtanga vinyasa* yoga, while Krishnamacharya's son, T.K.V. Desikachar followed his more gentle later teachings to develop *viniyoga*: healing yoga sequences tailored to suit individual needs. Krishnamacharya's first woman (and first Western) student, Indra Devi (1899–2002), also went on to make hatha yoga accessible to people across the world.

Swami Sivananda (1887–1963) developed his spiritually infused hatha yoga in Rishikesh, northern India, where disciples came to study the yoga path. One of them, Swami Vishnu Devananda (1927–93), left India for San Francisco in the 1950s, taking with him the form of yoga that inspires one of the largest worldwide schools of yoga, and which shows how to integrate the principles of the eight-fold path into modern life.

>> **Patanjali's** eightfold yoga path

The first five "limbs" below are practiced together and bring about the final three.

- **1 Yama**, social disciplines of conduct, urge us to be truthful, use sexual energy well, and not harm, steal, or be greedy.

- **2 Niyama**, individual disciplines of conduct, advise certain cleansing practices and spiritual austerities, as well as being content, undertaking self-study, and devotion to God.

- **3 Asana**, the physical postures we think of as yoga are but one part, intended to make the body stable and the mind poised.

- **4 Pranayama**, the breathing practices we encounter in yoga class, help keep the life-force in constant motion.

- **5 Pratyahara**, exercises to consciously withdraw the senses, foster tranquillity.

- **6 Dharana**, techniques to cultivate concentration on one point, lead to limb 7.

- **7 Dhyana**, uninterrupted focus, or meditation, leads to the final limb.

- **8 Samadhi**, a sense of oneness and peace.

>> **adapting** your lifestyle

A traditional yogic lifestyle is built around five principles: proper relaxation, proper exercise, proper breathing, proper diet, and positive thinking and meditation. Here are some ways to bring them into your own life, which is often as easy as living more simply.

You don't have to retreat to a mountaintop or move out of the city to live your life according to yogic principles. The simplest way to introduce them into your life and home is to let go of a consumer approach to living and to let an awareness of the planet and all those who share it inform the way you work, play, eat, and shop, which helps to bring your priorities into balance.

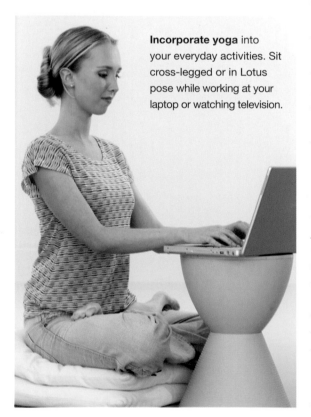

Incorporate yoga into your everyday activities. Sit cross-legged or in Lotus pose while working at your laptop or watching television.

Living a relaxed life

Relaxing is more than setting aside time to relax by meditating or going for a massage—though these are helpful for stress-recovery—it's about finding a lifestyle that nourishes you and allows you time to spend with the people you love and in the places that inspire you. If current commitments have you working all hours and racing from place to place, you need to sit down and think about how you might simplify things. Could you opt for part-time work, perhaps, work flexibly or from home sometimes? Once the basics are in place, look at ways of introducing more relaxing pursuits into your day. Build in times to listen to beautiful music, watch inspiring films, and read uplifting books; keep a CD in the car to sing along to; book a yoga vacation or weekend break; and, most importantly, make space for simply sitting in silence doing nothing every day.

"Proper exercising" isn't something you only do at yoga class; it's about using your muscles and joints as they were meant to be used every day (which wasn't by moving only from car to office chair to sofa). Try to make your life more active by choosing to walk whenever possible rather than using transportation, and take regular breaks from work to stretch out. Make sure the activities you use to relax are based around a good amount of activity, too—gardening, walking, and dancing are perfect.

We learn "proper breathing" of course, as we practice yoga's *pranayama* exercises, but this pillar of yogic balance also encourages us to be aware of

>> who are you?

- **You are what you think**, yoga teaches, so reflect on your thoughts as you go about your day, and observe how they color your reactions to events and people.

- **Respect yourself** first in order to learn how to respect others. You can do this by becoming aware of your negative self-talk and by taking steps to replace it with positive affirmations (see p121).

- **"Are you friend material?"** yoga encourages us to ask. It's good to keep thinking about how you might become the kind of person you would like as a friend.

- **How creative are you?** Yoga encourages creative pursuits to keep the mind vibrant.

At work and at home there are plenty of ways to become more active, from practicing leg raises during phone calls to conducting meetings on a walk.

our breathing in everyday situations. Bring your attention to your breath especially when you feel anxious (see p122), watching it become slower and deeper. This results in a calm mind, too.

We are what we eat

A diet rich in *sattwic* foods—those bursting with vitality, such as fresh, seasonal fruit and vegetables and whole grains—nourishes the body with vitamins and minerals, keeps the mind relaxed and the emotions steady. But what we eat has an ethical dimension that can nourish the spirit, too. Building your diet around local, seasonal produce cuts down on food-transportation miles that have a detrimental effect on our planet, and choosing fairly traded goods from abroad and products from small suppliers near to home ensures that consumption reflects your yogic principles. Some people who practice yoga extend the *yama* of nonviolence (see p117) to diet, choosing not to eat meat.

Honor the origins of the foodstuffs you buy by cooking them with care, and by sharing them with those you love, giving thanks before you eat.

>> **positive** thinking

The last of the five principles of the yoga lifestyle, positive thinking and meditation, encourages us to look at our habitual reactions and train the mind to respond in ways more beneficial to well-being and peace. Steps to simple meditation and relaxed breathing are on pages 122–23.

If you feel joyous and full of positive energy, you will find that the people you mix with brighten up—and when we laugh, life seems less onerous and distressing, and the body's systems, including immune and nervous function, work more effectively. Yoga teaches the art of turning negative thinking into more positive thought patterns. Its methods are gentle and begin by showing us how to become aware of our current predilections. Try it out by spending a minute or two after you wake

observing how you feel. Is your glass half full or half empty this morning? Having gained this information, try not to judge yourself, which can set up a thought-train of negativity and self-loathing. Instead, reflect on how it might encourage others to react to you as the day goes on. Feel responsible

To make yourself more comfortable in the relaxation pose, place an eye pad over your eyes, a firm bolster under your knees, and cushion your neck and ankles.

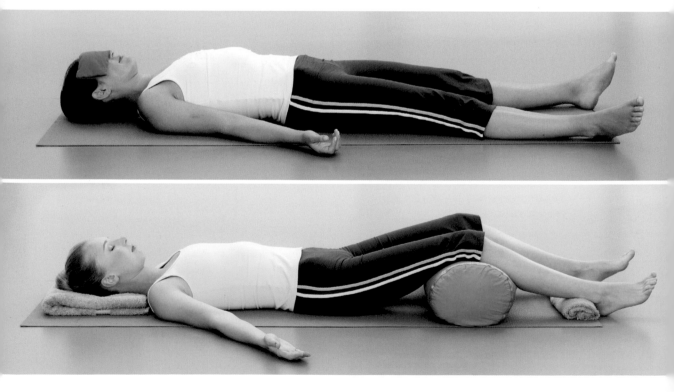

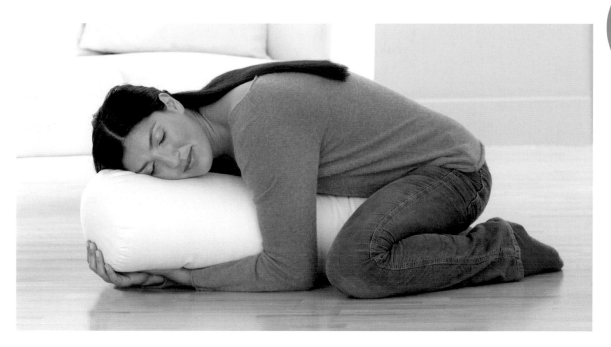

for yourself and the way in which your behavior will influence your future and the lives of those you interact with today. Then gently encourage your mind to be as open to positivity as it can be. It may help to make an affirmation—a positive statement in the first person and the present tense—and to repeat it beneath your breath like a mantra. Choose words that encourage you to lighten up and let go of anxiety. You might say, "I feel open and happy" or, "I feel ready to respond to today's challenges with relaxed positivity."

Relaxation pose

Spending time in yoga relaxation postures can support your efforts toward positivity—letting go of your body and your thoughts in Corpse pose needn't be reserved for the end of a yoga class. Drop into this pose any time you would like to counter negativity or feel in need of a little positive nurturing by lying on your back with your legs apart and feet flopping outward and your arms away from your sides, palms facing upward and fingers gently curled (top, opposite). Yoga teaches that the mind becomes more settled and balanced when the body is aligned symmetrically in rest. If you are pregnant, lie on your side with pillows behind your

Grab opportunities to relax as you move through the day. You don't need to adopt the formal Corpse pose: sitting on your heels and relaxing forward onto cushions for a few minutes helps you maintain equanimity and positivity.

back and under your upper leg. To bring about a deep state of relaxation more quickly, cover your eyes with an eye pad, and let its heaviness encourage you to allow all five senses to retreat deep within.

Although this pose of positive relaxation may appear easy, it is notoriously difficult to master, since it asks you not only to still every part of your body, but to gaze within at the "monkey mind," which jumps from thought to scattered thought, and may dwell on negativity. It can also be tempting simply to drift off, a common experience when you first start yoga. Don't beat yourself up. If you practice this relaxation pose regularly—for five to 20 minutes every day—your body will sink into ease more effectively and your mind will remain simultaneously more relaxed and more alert as you become a detached observer, standing aside to watch your body and breath become completely relaxed. There follows a peaceful, naturally joyous, calm mind that equips us to ride stressful situations and carry positive vibes out into the world.

>> meditation

Meditating helps you to achieve inner and outer harmony, to feel alive, and at peace. Once you get into the habit of meditating, it becomes a part of you. Watching your breath (*pranayama*) helps you keep focused and become aware if you are pushing yourself too far in your practice.

Use meditation to clean your mind. We clean our bodies, teeth, clothes, and home, but often ignore our inner self as if it does not exist. It takes discipline and is not easy, but like everything, you have to practice to reap the benefits.

How to meditate

Set aside a certain amount of time each day to meditate. It helps if it is the same time each day; early morning or early evening are good times, but choose a time that fits in with your lifestyle. Try to meditate in the same place each day. Find a quiet corner in your home, where you can create a peaceful atmosphere. Light a candle or place a bowl of flowers or a picture of someone who inspires you there.

You can meditate sitting in a chair or on the floor—whatever feels best. If you choose to sit on a chair, use a comfortable, upright chair and sit on it with your back straight, not leaning on the back. Place your feet firmly on the floor with your hands resting on your thighs. You can either kneel or sit cross-legged on the floor. Choose one position to sit in for the whole period. Sit up straight on a cushion or two.

Set a timer and sit still, watching your breath, repeating a word, or holding a vision in your mind. Be kind to yourself because it is not as easy as it sounds. Do not be too ambitious to begin with. Set a manageable amount of time aside for you to sit there, with all your thoughts and discomforts, and keep on returning to that simple breath, mantra, or inner vision. Sit still, even if you feel discomfort, pain, itchiness, and restlessness, coming back to your focus point every time you notice you have wandered off. When the timer goes off, even if you want to stay longer, finish there, and repeat the same every day, slowly building up to about 30 minutes of meditation once or twice a day. After regularly meditating for about a month, you may notice that you are calmer and that you feel more spaciousness in your life.

Pranayama

Your best friend in yoga is your breath. You should be watching your breath in the background constantly as you practice. People who are new to yoga are very often shallow breathers. Becoming aware of this is a significant first step. It is important to let the breath flow freely while performing the postures. As a beginner, you are not trying to control the breath, but just getting to know it as it is. If the breath becomes labored and shaky, this means you are going too far. Watching your breath is a great monitor and focus point to prevent your mind from wandering onto everyday matters while you are practicing. Your breath can lead your mind to parts of the body that are asking for special attention and, over time, you can learn to release tensions and blockages with the help of your breath.

Meditate in comfortable, relaxing surroundings. Sit cross-legged, on a chair, or kneel, placing your hands on your lap or resting on your thighs.

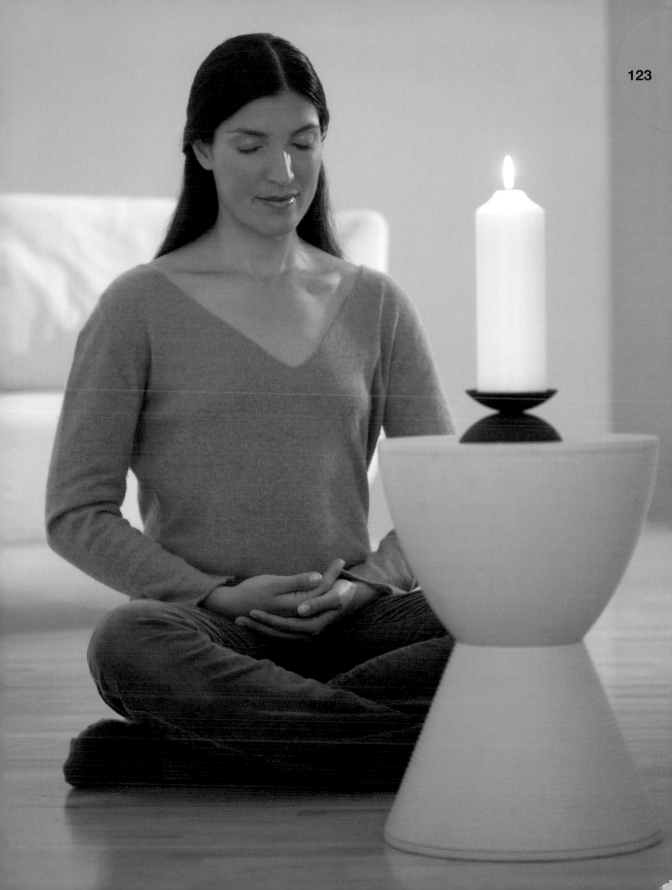

useful resources

Consult the following list of organizations and websites to help you to find a class or meditation center, stockists of equipment and clothing, and to book a retreat or holiday. If you want to find out more about yoga, see the recommended reading list to help you further on your yogic path.

United States

Finding a teacher

When you are ready take a yoga class or be part of a larger learning community, it's important to find a place where you feel welcome and at ease.

BKS Iyengar Yoga National Association of the United States

www.iynaus.org
tel: 800 889-YOGA
Search for certified Iyengar yoga teachers by state, become a member, and access links of yoga resources.

Yoga Alliance

www.yogaalliance.org
tel: 877-964-2255
Find a Yoga Alliance certified teacher or yoga center through this national Yoga Teacher's Registry.

Yoga Finder

www.yogafinder.com
tel: 858-213-7924
Locate teachers and classes of all types of yoga along with equipment and event resources.

Equipment and clothing

Hugger Mugger Yoga Products

www.huggermugger.com
tel: 800-473-4888
Stable, non-slip mats and clothing available for wholesale or retail.

Manduka

www.manduka.com
tel: 805-544-3744
High-performance, ecologically friendly mats, bags, towels, accessories, and apparel.

Prana

www.prana.com
tel: 800-557-7262
Clothing and leisure wear from outdoors apparel company.

Saka

www.sakayoga.com
tel: 802-660-4889
Yoga bags, totes, and accessories for integrating life off and on the mat.

Yoga Props

www.yogaprops.com
tel: 888-856-9642
Offers a wide selection of mats, blocks, bags, straps, etc.

Retreats and holidays

Himalyan Institute

www.himalayaninstitute.org
tel: 800-822-4547
Headquartered in rural Pennsylvania, the center offers programs in hatha yoga, meditation, stress reduction, Ayurveda, nutrition, spirituality, and Eastern philosophy.

Kripalu Center for Yoga and Health

www.kripalu.org
tel: 866-200-5203
Retreat center in New England with everything from great yoga classes to massages. Kripalu hosts famous teachers in yoga, Buddhism, and other contemplative arts.

Omega Institute

www.eomega.org
tel: 800-944-1001
Retreats and workshops in Rhinebeck, New York, and winter programs in warmer climates.

Meditation

Shambhala Mountain Center

4921 County Road, 68-C Red Feather Lakes, Colorado 80545
www.shambhalamountain.org
tel: 1-888-STUPA-21 (788-7221)
A mountain valley retreat offering programs on Buddhist meditation and yoga.

Friends of the Western Buddhist Order

www.fwbo.org
Find information on how to meditate and details on FWBO centers' locations and activities across the world.

The World Community for Christian Meditation

www.wccm.org
tel: +44 (0)207 278 2070
Find information on meditation, groups, and centers.

Recommended reading

Find out more about different styles of yoga, meditation, breathing, and the benefits of yoga, and learn how to incorporate yoga into your life.

Anatomy of Hatha Yoga
H. David Coulter
Body and Breath, Inc.
Comprehensive resource relating the mechanics of the body to yoga.

The Bhagavad Gita
There are thousands of versions of this available. An easy one to start with is *Perennial Psychology of the Bhagavad Gita*

by Swami Rama; Himalayan Institute Press.

The Breathing Book: Vitality and Good Health Through Essential Breath Work
Donna Farhi
Holt (Henry) & Co

Bringing Yoga to Life
Donna Farhi
HarperCollins

Easy Does It Yoga
Alice Christensen
Fireside Books

The Heart of Yoga
T.K.V. Desikachar
Inner Traditions International

How to Use Yoga: A Step-by-step Guide to the Iyengar Method of Yoga, for Relaxation, Health and Well-being
Mira Mehta
Southwater

Keep It Simple Series (KISS)
Guide to Yoga
Shakta Kaur Khalsa
DK Publishing

Light on Yoga: The Bible of Modern Yoga—Its Philosophy and Practice—by the World's Foremost Teacher
B.K.S. Iyengar
Schocken Books

Mindfulness Bliss and Beyond: A Meditator's Handbook
Ajahn Brahm
Wisdom Publications
Patanjali's Yoga Sutras

Try *How to Know God* by Swami Prabhavananda and Christopher Isherwood; Vedanta Centre Publishers

Yoga Body, Buddha Mind
Cyndi Lee
Riverhead Books

Yoga For Life
Margaret and Martin Pierce
Sterling Publishing

Yoga: Path to Holistic Health
B.K.S. Iyengar
Dorling Kindersley

Yoga: the Iyengar Way
Mira Silva and Mehta Shyam
Dorling Kindersley

Yoga Mind, Body and Spirit: A Return to Wholeness
Donna Farhi
Newleaf

Canada

Finding a teacher

Yoga in Canada
www.yogadirectorycanada.com
tel: (514) 341-4457
Find a yoga class, teacher or studio, as well as a list of retreats and yoga resources.

Equipment and clothing

Lululemon
www.lululemon.com
tel: (877) 263-9300
Yoga and athletic clothing and accessories for women and men.

index

acknowledgments

Author's acknowledgments

Thank you to everyone who made this project possible: Helen Murray, my editor, who was always there encouraging me, and Anne Fisher, the designer, who made it all look so beautiful; Ruth Jenkinson for her exquisite photography; all at Chrome Productions, especially Gez, Hannah, and Sami, for the DVD. What would I have done without Susan Reynolds and Tara Lee, the models, who were brilliant and so supportive behind the scenes? Thank you also to Penny Warren and Mary-Clare Jerram for instigating the project and all the behind-the-scenes DK staff who helped to pull it all together. A big thank you to Rebekah Hay Brown, Anna Blackmore, and Anne Manderson, who were always at the end of the phone and ready to pop round at the drop of a hat. Not to forget all the students I teach, who give me so much joy and who I learn so much from. Lastly, and most importantly of all, my wonderful husband, Richard Brown.

Publisher's acknowledgments

Dorling Kindersley would like to thank photographer Ruth Jenkinson and her assistants, James McNaught and Vic Churchill; sweatyBetty for the loan of the exercise clothing; Viv Riley at Touch Studios; the models Tara Lee and Susan Reynolds; Roisin Donaghy and Victoria Barnes for the hair and makeup; Claire Tennant-Scull for proofreading and Hilary Bird for compiling the index with very limited time. A special thanks to YogaMatters for the loan of the mat and other equipment. Lastly, thanks to Susannah Marriott for her expert editorial assistance.

Picture credits

The publisher would like to thank the following for their kind permission to reproduce their photographs: Krishnamacharya Yoga Mandiram: 116; Sivananda Yoga Vedanta Centers: 117.
All other images © Dorling Kindersley
For further information see: www.dkimages.com

about Louise Grime

Louise teaches hatha yoga in London, mainly at triyoga in Primrose Hill and Soho and at The Life Centre, Notting Hill Gate. She started practicing yoga with Silvia Prescott and Penny Neild-Smith, two of the first Iyengar teachers in London, in 1978. Since then, she has spent time in the Sivananda Ashram in Kerala, India, where she completed teachers' training and advanced teachers' training. In 1994, Louise qualified as an Iyengar yoga teacher in London and then met Shandor Remete who introduced her to Shadow Yoga. In the 90s, she practiced Ashtanga Vinyasa Yoga with John Scott. Louise takes a keen interest in Eastern and Western spiritual traditions and meditation. When teaching she likes to incorporate the yogic philosophy into her classes. She is one of the teachers on The Life Centre's Level 1 Teacher Training Programme. Louise has also worked as a journalist, restaurant manager, and as a stage manager in theatre and television.